Urology

£1.50

Urology

JOHN BLANDY
CBE, MA, DM, MCh, FRCS, FACS, (Hon) FRCSI
Emeritus Professor of Urology,
University of London
at the London Hospital Medical College;
Consulting Urologist, St Peter's Hospital

Fifth edition

b

Blackwell
Science

© 1976, 1977, 1982, 1989, 1998 by
Blackwell Science Ltd
Editorial Offices:
Osney Mead, Oxford OX2 0EL
25 John Street, London WC1N 2BL
23 Ainslie Place, Edinburgh EH3 6AJ
350 Main Street, Malden
 MA 02148 5018, USA
54 University Street, Carlton
 Victoria 3053, Australia
10, rue Casimir Delavigne
 75006 Paris, France

Other Editorial Offices:
Blackwell Wissenschafts-Verlag GmbH
Kurfürstendamm 57
10707 Berlin, Germany

Blackwell Science KK
MG Kodenmacho Building
7–10 Kodenmacho Nihombashi
Chuo-ku, Tokyo 104, Japan

The right of the Author to be identified as
the Author of this Work has been asserted in
accordance with the Copyright, Designs and
Patents Act 1988.

Set by Excel Typesetters Co., Hong Kong
Printed and bound in the United Kingdom at
the University Press, Cambridge

A catalogue record for this title
is available from the British Library

ISBN 0-632-04202-8

Library of Congress
Cataloging-in-Publication Data

Blandy, John P. (John Peter), 1927–
  Lecture notes on urology/John Blandy.
  —5th ed.
     p.   cm.
  Includes bibliographical references
and index.
  ISBN 0-632-04202-8
  1. Urinary organs — Diseases —
Outlines, syllabi, etc.
  2. Urology — Outlines, syllabi, etc.
  I. Title
  [DNLM: I. Urologic Diseases.
WJ 140 B642L 1998]
RC900.5.B53   1998
616.6—dc21
DNLM/DLC
for Library of Congress   97-23639
                                         CIP

First published 1976
Second edition 1977
Reprinted 1979
Third edition 1982
Reprinted 1984, 1986, 1988
Fourth edition 1989
Fifth edition 1998
Reprinted 1999

DISTRIBUTORS

 Marston Book Services Ltd
 PO Box 269
 Abingdon, Oxon OX14 4YN
 (Orders: Tel: 01235 465500
         Fax: 01235 465555)

USA
 Blackwell Science, Inc.
 Commerce Place
 350 Main Street
 Malden, MA 02148 5018
 (Orders: Tel: 800 759 6102
          781 388 8250
     Fax: 781 388 8255)

Canada
 Login Brothers Book Company
 324 Saulteaux Crescent
 Winnipeg, Manitoba R3J 3T2
 (Orders: Tel: 204 837 2987)

Australia
 Blackwell Science Pty Ltd
 54 University Street
 Carlton, Victoria 3053
 (Orders: Tel: 03 9347 0300
         Fax: 03 9347 5001)

The Blackwell Science logo is a trade mark of
Blackwell Science Ltd, registered at the
United Kingdom Trade Marks Registry

For further information on
Blackwell Science, visit our website:
www.blackwell-science.com

Contents

Preface to the Fifth Edition

Urology has seen many changes in the time since the previous edition was revised, and it has once more been necessary to rewrite it almost entirely, taking the opportunity to drop some things that have become out of date and introduce much that is new and exciting. Thanks largely to the pace of technological change, there have been so many innovations that it is not always easy to distinguish the truly useful from the passing craze.

At no time has urology not been an essential part of the work of the doctor, but the medical undergraduate's curriculum is today so crowded that it becomes even more necessary to prune away those matters which are probably only relevant to the trainee surgeon. As for the list of jargon and eponyms, this was never necessary, but remains, if somewhat truncated, just for fun.

J.P.B.

Preface to the First Edition

This book has been written for the undergraduate medical student. About a quarter of all the operations of surgery concern the genitourinary system: about 15% of all doctors suffer at some time or other from a stone in the urinary tract: one in ten of all males has to have an operation on his prostate before he reaches the end of his days. The management of haematuria, of impotence, of infertility, and of urinary tract infections: the investigation of hypertension, and the evaluation of albuminuria — no doctor, however recondite his specialty, is not at some time touched by one or other of these common problems. Of all diseases in the world, in prevalence second only to malaria, schistosomiasis affects more human beings, and those more miserably, than any other. The author makes no apology therefore for the claim that the specialty of urology encompasses some of the most important, and arguably the most fascinating of all the topics of medicine and surgery. My object has been to communicate my own interest and enthusiasm to my students, for unlike some topics which they have to learn, there ought to be nothing boring or dull in this, the oldest and most vigorous of all the specialties. It is for this reason that the solemn minded reader may not approve of some of my pictures, or my omission of the customary protracted dissertation about body fluids and electrolytes for which he will have to consult those of his textbooks which deal with them in a way which I could not imitate even if I understood. Sexually transmitted diseases are not covered in this book, not because I find them tedious, but because they are too important to be dealt with by other than an expert. On the other hand I found it impossible not to trespass from time to time on the ground normally and correctly assigned to my colleagues in nephrology from whom I crave forgiveness if, in an attempt to make an understandable and unified presentation of the subject, my ignorance has led me into too many and too barbarous errors concerning the esoteric mysteries of nephritis and hypertension. The last chapter about the operations of urology is there simply to make the students' visits to the operating theatre more interesting: they should not attempt to learn surgical technique—though I hope they may find watching operations helps in the understanding of living pathology. For the same reason the little glossary of jargon, eponyms and gobbledegook is added for fun, not because students need learn any of it.

J.P.B.

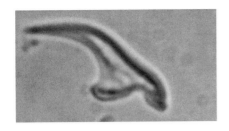

History and Examination

Begin at the beginning: how old is your patient and what is his or her occupation? Do they smoke? Have they travelled in Africa or Indochina? Ask retired people about their previous occupation especially if there was any exposure to rubber, chemicals or plastics. Women should be asked how many and how old are their children, and whether there was any complication during pregnancy or delivery that may have required a catheter, which might have introduced infection.

What brings the patient to you? What were the first symptoms? When did they begin: and how did they change as time went by? Let the patient do the talking — listening is the key to taking a history. Try to get a clear picture of the way the illness developed over the years, and make sure you really understand just what is bothering him or her right now. Never end your enquiry without asking whether the patient has noticed blood in the urine: haematuria is the single most important symptom in the whole of urology.

Your notes should be brief, but sufficiently clear that if you drop dead, another doctor can take up management of the case. No note is of any use if it cannot be read. If your handwriting is really bad, teach yourself to use a word-processor. Put the date and name of the patient on every page. Your notes are now available to the patient and may at any time be used as evidence in a court of law, so be polite about your patient and loyal to your colleagues: never be tempted to make an unfair or disparaging criticism of a professional colleague.

A drawing can save many words, so a sketch noting where the pain starts from and radiates to would be useful, together with a word or two to specify the type of pain, e.g. sharp, colicky, dull, etc. (Fig. 1.1).

Avoid pretentious Greek or Latin terms unless they are clear and unambiguous. Dysuria can mean pain or difficulty or both: which do you really mean? Frequency is expressed by writing down how often your patient voids by day and by night, e.g. D = 6, N = 3. Enuresis can be ambiguous: if you mean the patient wets the bed, why not say so?

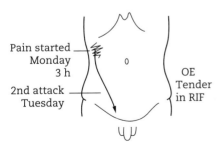

Pain started
Monday
3 h

2nd attack
Tuesday

0

OE
Tender
in RIF

Fig. 1.1 A sketch showing the main features in a patient with right ureteric colic.

An exception is the term haematuria. It matters little whether the blood has been seen by the patient or found in a stix test, nor whether it is well mixed or appears at the beginning or the end of the stream: any kind of blood in the urine demands a thorough investigation. Blood trickling from the urethra between acts of urination is probably coming from the urethra, but it still needs investigation.

PREVIOUS HISTORY

Ask about rheumatism and arthritis for which analgesics may have been taken: analgesic nephropathy is surprisingly common and seldom suspected unless you ask about the consumption of pain-killing tablets.

Students often feel awkward when asking about venereal disease. In times past men were usually secretly flattered at the suggestion that they might have been a Don Juan when young: today one must be aware of the possibility of acquired immune deficiency syndrome (AIDS).

Do not waste time. As you listen to the patient it may be obvious that certain investigations are going to be needed. Unobtrusively filling in the relevant forms will not stop you listening politely but will save time, and more importantly, may prevent you from writing down too much. Listening is far more important than writing.

PHYSICAL EXAMINATION

Physical examination begins as the patient comes into the room. Does the patient look ill? Has the patient obviously lost weight? Does the gait suggest pain, parkinsonism or ankylosing spondylitis? Is there that faint whiff of urine that suggests uraemia, or the frank ammoniacal reek of wet trousers?

To rise to shake your patient's hand is not mere politeness: it gives useful information. Whatever your specialty, never forget that you are a doctor first and your concern is for the patient as a whole. In an ideal world, where no doctor was ever pushed for time and no patient ever in a hurry to get back to work or children, you could spend all day over one case, getting to know your patient in depth and making a thorough and complete physical examination of every system. Something approaching such a thorough clerking is indeed necessary when admitting a patient to the ward, but in the outpatient clinic it would be cruelly slow and unfair to the others who are waiting. Of course, if you do notice something that draws attention to a disorder in another system, by all means examine that system as well.

In most patients who attend the urological clinic you are looking for enlargement of a kidney or bladder, disorders in the inguinal region or genitalia, hypertension, and signs in the pelvis that might be detected by vaginal or rectal examination. It is to these features that you should chiefly direct your attention.

ABDOMINAL EXAMINATION

The traditional physical signs of an enlarged kidney (Fig. 1.2) are a rounded lump in the loin, bimanually palpable, moving on respiration. You can get your hand between the lump and the edge of the costal margin. There is said to be a band of resonance in front of the kidney due to gas in the bowel (Fig. 1.3). None of these physical signs is trustworthy: on the right side the supposed 'kidney' may turn out to be the gall bladder or liver, and on the left it may prove to be the spleen, even though you think you can slide your hand between the lump and the costal margin. A large mass may arise from or displace the colon.

An enlarged bladder (Figs 1.4, 1.5) may be equally misleading. One expects to find a rounded swelling arising out of the pelvis which is dull to percussion. In practice a floppy, over-distended bladder may be so soft that it is difficult to feel, and the bladder does not always rise up as it ought to do, in the midline, but often is more to one side than the other. The infallible sign is that the swelling goes away if you let the urine out with a catheter.

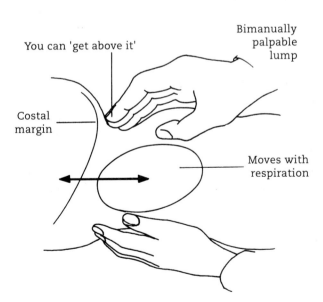

Fig. 1.2 Physical signs of an enlarged kidney.

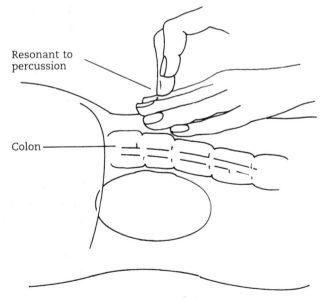

Fig. 1.3 There is often a band of resonance in front of the kidney from gas in the colon.

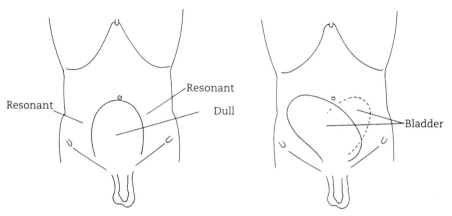

Fig. 1.4 The bladder is dull to percussion.   **Fig. 1.5** An enlarging bladder may go to one or other side.

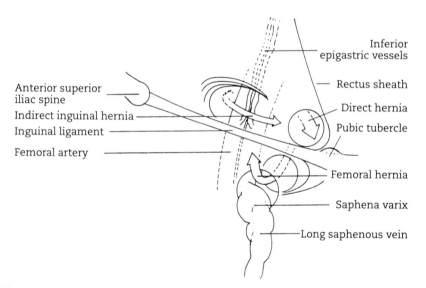

Fig. 1.6 Landmarks for groin hernias.

Examination of the inguinal regions is concerned with three hernial orifices on each side (Fig. 1.6). Each must be felt with the patient standing up, lying down, and coughing.

1   An indirect inguinal hernia emerges lateral to the inferior epigastric vessels and slides down the inguinal canal to the scrotum.

2   A direct inguinal hernia emerges medial to the inferior epigastric vessels, and seldom enters the scrotum.

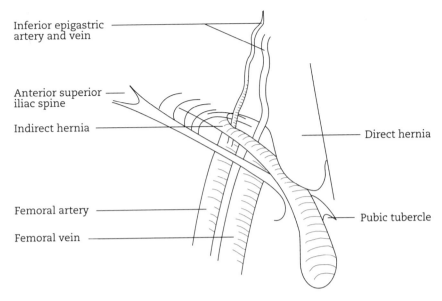

Fig. 1.7 Pantaloon hernia.

Direct and indirect inguinal herniae may be present in the same patient, with the two sacs emerging like a pair of trousers on either side of the inferior epigastric vessels (Fig. 1.7).

3 A femoral hernia pushes out below the inguinal ligament, medial to the femoral vein, and then bulges up and out through the gap in the deep fascia where the saphenous vein joins the femoral vein. The sac has a narrow neck, and is always surrounded by layer upon layer of fat like an onion, so that a cough impulse can be difficult to feel. A femoral hernia is mimicked by a saphena varix, the dilated upper end of the saphenous vein, but this has a cough thrill which runs down the saphenous vein, and the lump disappears when the patient lies down.

THE SCROTUM AND ITS CONTENTS

The term 'testicle' includes testis and epididymis. When examining the scrotum the first thing to make sure of is that the swelling is not a hernia, i.e. coming down along the spermatic cord from above. Ask yourself the following simple questions:

1 Can you 'get above' the swelling? If you can, it must be in the testicle (Fig. 1.8).

2 Is the lump fluctuant? Verify this by testing in two planes (Fig. 1.9). If it is fluctuant, then:

(a) is it in front of the testis? If so, it is a hydrocele—fluid in the sac of the tunica vaginalis (see. p. 261) (Fig. 1.10);

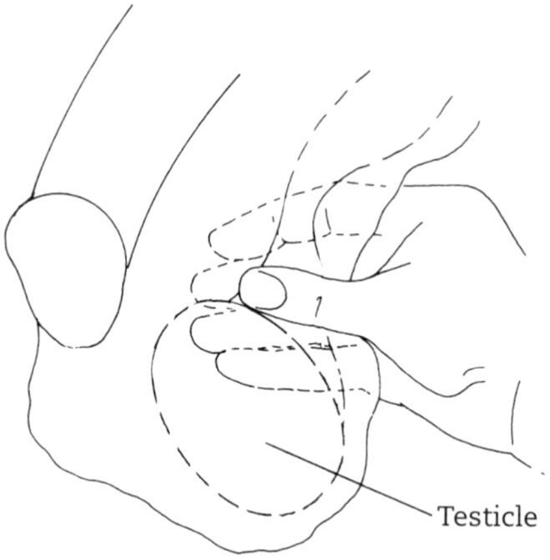

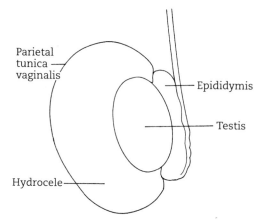

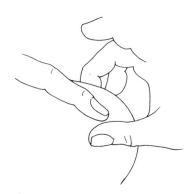

Fig. 1.8 Lump in the scrotum: can you get above it?

Fig. 1.9 Lump in the scrotum: check whether it is solid or fluctuant. Determine fluctuation in two planes.

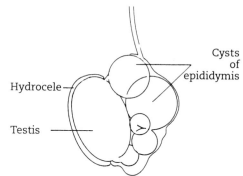

Fig. 1.10 Hydroceles lie in front of the testis and tend to surround it.

Fig. 1.11 Cystic swellings behind the testis are cysts of the epididymis.

(b)   is it behind the testis? If so, it is a collection of cysts of the epididymis (see p. 262) (Fig. 1.11); or

(c)   can you shine a light through it? An empty cylinder makes it easier to be sure of this in a well-lit room (Fig. 1.12). If light does not shine through the swelling, either the wall of the swelling is thickened, or it contains not innocent clear fluid, but pus, blood or cancer.

3   If the lump is not fluctuant, i.e. is solid, decide whether it is arising from the testis or the epididymis:

(a)   a solid lump arising from the testis is cancer until proved otherwise (see p. 266) (Fig. 1.13);

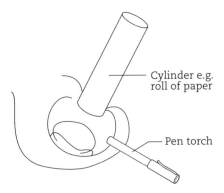

Fig. 1.12 To see if light shines through a swelling it helps to use a cylinder, e.g. one made from a rolled-up paper.

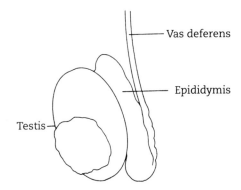

Fig. 1.13 A solid swelling in the testis is a cancer until proved otherwise.

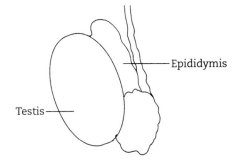

Fig. 1.14 Solid swellings in the epididymis are usually inflammatory.

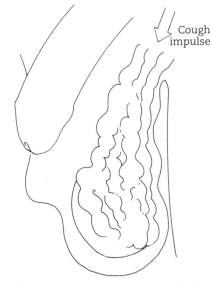

Fig. 1.15 Varicocele: enlarged testicular veins. There is a cough impulse and the swelling disappears when the patient lies down.

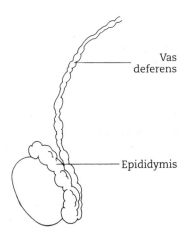

Fig. 1.16 Multiple knotty swellings in the epididymis and vas are typical of tuberculosis.

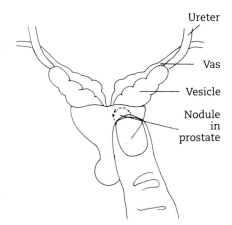

Fig. 1.17 Anatomical landmarks that may be felt per rectum.

(b)   a solid lump arising from the epididymis is usually benign, but calls for further investigation (see p. 265) (Fig. 1.14).

SWELLINGS IN THE SPERMATIC CORD

VARICOCELE
The veins draining the testicle may become varicose and distended, feeling like a 'bag of worms', and there is a cough impulse (Fig. 1.15). (Like you, I have never actually felt a bag of worms, but we both know what it would feel like.)

VAS DEFERENS
The vas deferens lies posterior to the spermatic cord. If the vas is inflamed or has been operated on, e.g. by vasectomy, one may feel nodules along its course. Multiple knotty swellings are typical of tuberculosis (Fig. 1.16) and inflammatory swellings in the cord are seen in the tropical conditions of schistosomiasis and filariasis (see p. 265).

RECTAL EXAMINATION

One may perform a rectal examination in either sex in the supine, knee–elbow or left lateral position. Always introduce your finger slowly and gently to allow the sphincter to relax (everyone knows the need to pass a constipated stool slowly). Once inside the rectum feel the prostate and the rest of the wall of the rectum carefully—you will sometimes detect an entirely unexpected cancer of the rectum (Fig. 1.17).

Feel the prostate carefully for hardness or nodules which may mean cancer (see p. 205). Even if it feels normal, try to estimate its size. If the prostate is tender on light palpation, it may be the site of inflammation (see p. 193). Mistakes are easy to make when performing a rectal examination, but the worst mistake is not to do one at all.

FURTHER READING

Blandy JP, Fowler CG (1996) *Urology*, 2nd edn. Oxford, Blackwell Science.
Frecchia JA, Motta J, Miller LS, Armenakas NA, Schumann GB, Greenberg RA (1995) Evaluation of asymptomatic microhematuria. *Urology* **46**: 484.
Nunns D, Smith ARB, Hosker G (1995) Reagent strip testing urine for significant bacteriuria in a urodynamic clinic. *Br J Urol* **76**: 87.

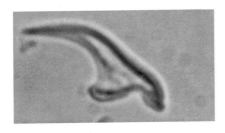

Investigations

TESTING THE URINE

For centuries the doctor has learnt much from the urine: in times past the doctor would look at it, measure it, smell it and even taste it. Today he or she need not taste it but the other senses are still useful. Infected urine usually stinks, and it is always cloudy. Crystal clear urine is never infected. On many occasions a diagnosis may be made by having the patient simply record the time and volume of urine passed during 24 h—the voiding diary or urine output chart (Fig. 2.1).

OFFICE TESTS OF THE URINE

pH
Indicator dyes impregnated on a paper strip measure pH sufficiently accurately for most purposes. Very acid urine should make you suspect uric acid stones (see p. 76). Very alkaline urine suggests infection with a microorganism that splits urea, e.g. *Proteus mirabilis*.

PROTEIN
1 Paper strips impregnated with tetrabromophenol normally turn blue in the pH range found in normal urine. Protein makes the colour yellowish. The dye is an indicator, and is not reliable in extremes of acidity or alkalinity.
2 A more reliable test for protein is to add a drop of 25% salicylsulphonic acid: this precipitates protein as a cloud unless the urine is exceptionally dilute.

7.30 am	300	cc	Tuesday
8.15 "	150	cc	
11.10 "	100	cc	
12.35 pm	150	cc	
2.00 "	150	cc	
4.30 "	150	cc	
6.30 "	175	cc	
8.00 "	175	cc	
11.00 "	150	cc	
7.00 am	250	cc	Wednesday

Fig. 2.1 Voiding diary or fluid output chart.

3 Boiling the urine precipitates a cloud, which persists when you add a drop of a dilute acid. If the cloud disappears, it was due to phosphates.

4 When it is essential to know whether the quantity of protein in the urine is significant, collect the urine over 24 h and have the protein measured quantitatively in the laboratory: more than 150 mg protein per 24 h is abnormal and requires further investigation (see p. 57).

GLUCOSE

1 Paper strips are impregnated with glucose oxidase, an enzyme which converts glucose to gluconic acid and hydrogen peroxide. The paper also contains peroxidase which catalyses the reaction between hydrogen peroxide and potassium iodide to give a green–brown colour.

2 When paper strips are unavailable, boil the urine with Fehling's or Benedict's solution. Glucose and other reducing substances throw down an orange precipitate of copper.

BLOOD IN THE URINE

Commercial stix tests for haematuria rely on the oxidation of tetramethylbenzidine by cumene peroxidase, which is catalysed by haemoglobin to give a green–blue colour. Bear in mind that you are testing for free haemoglobin. If the test is positive, examine the urine under a microscope to see if red cells are present (see below). The sensitivity of these stix tests is adjusted by the manufacturers to show a positive result when the amount of haemoglobin corresponds to about 10 red cells per high power field—twice the number found in normal urine — so a positive stix test always demands a thorough investigation (see p. 166).

False positive tests may occur if the glass container is contaminated with povidone iodine or has been cleaned with hypochlorite.

INFECTION

Office tests for infection are available that are based on bacterial conversion of nitrate to nitrite, or the detection of leucocytes by leucocyte esterase activity. They are of limited use (see p. 59).

BLADDER TUMOUR ANTIGEN

The Bard bladder tumour antigen (BTA) test is based on the fact that bladder tumours break down the basement membrane, and liberate a complex — bladder tumour antigen — that can be detected by latex particles coated with human immunoglobulin G. A specially prepared test strip produces a yellow band if positive, green if negative.

MICROSCOPIC EXAMINATION OF THE URINE

BLOOD

Put a drop of urine on a slide and cover with a cover-slip. More than 5 red cells per high power field is abnormal.

PUS

A similar drop of urine will show more than 5 white cells per high power field if there is infection. When the pus cells come from the kidney they have a characteristic glittering appearance. A Gram stain of the centrifuged deposit may identify the bacteria that are present.

CASTS

Casts are the squeezed-out contents of the collecting tubules of the kidney. When they are made of protein they are clear (hyaline): when made of red or white cells they are granular (Fig. 2.2).

CRYSTALS

In cool urine there are always some crystals of triple phosphate and calcium oxalate. The hexagonal plates of cystine give away the diagnosis of cystinuria (see p. 76). Uric acid crystals are specially common in acid urine (Fig. 2.3).

MYCOBACTERIUM TUBERCULOSIS

The centrifuged urine is stained with auramine and examined under ultraviolet light: the mycobacteria shine as bright yellow dots.

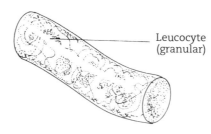
Protein (hyaline)

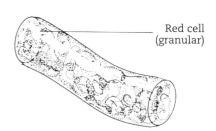
Leucocyte (granular)

Red cell (granular)

Fig. 2.2 Casts in the urine.

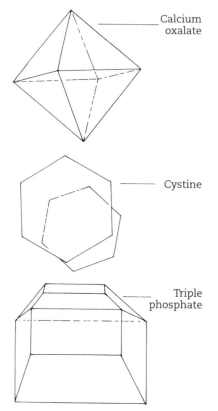
Calcium oxalate

Cystine

Triple phosphate

Fig. 2.3 Crystals in the urine.

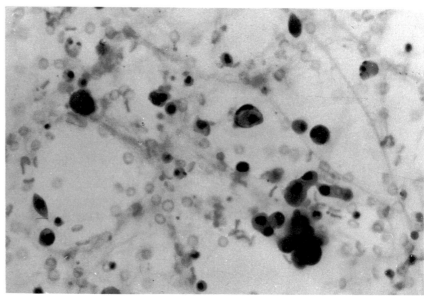

Fig. 2.4 Centrifuged deposit from urine stained to show cancer cells.

CANCER CELLS

The urine is fixed with a roughly equal volume of 10% formalin and sent to the laboratory where it is centrifuged: the deposit is made into a smear which is stained with methylene blue by Papanicolaou's method (Fig. 2.4). False negatives occur if the tumour is very well differentiated and sheds cells that are hardly different from normal urothelium. False positives occur if there has been recent injury, e.g. from the passage of a stone, when cells in mitosis because of normal healing may find their way into the urine.

SCHISTOSOMA OVA

The urine may show the characteristic ova of *Schistosoma haematobium* (see p. 158) (Fig. 2.5).

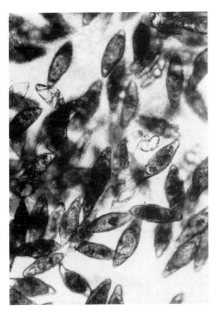

Fig. 2.5 Ova of *Schistosoma haematobium*.

CULTURE OF URINE

Urine is such an excellent culture medium that it is easily contaminated from the wall of the urethra, prepuce or vulva, and by air-borne dust. At room temperature these contaminants grow rapidly so that urine must either be plated out at once, or put in a refrigerator. It is all too easy to make a mistaken diagnosis of infection if the urine has been allowed to stand around at room temperature for a few hours before reaching the laboratory.

Even if cultured promptly, some of the organisms that appear in the urine will be contaminants, unless the urine has been obtained by needle aspiration from the bladder or from a catheter. Passing a catheter itself may introduce infection and is therefore avoided if possible, but it is (in theory) possible to distinguish between contaminants and truly infective organisms. If urine is mixed with a culture medium before incubation, each colony that grows must represent one organism, a colony count will give the numbers of bacteria present in the urine. In practice more than 50 000 (10^5) colonies/ml signifies infection, and anything less usually means contamination. Remember that these figures only apply to clean-voided urine. Any organisms that are found in urine obtained by direct aspiration or a catheter mean infection.

One easy way to make a colony-count is with a dip-slide (Fig. 2.6). Plastic slides coated with culture media are dipped in urine, drained off, placed in a sterile

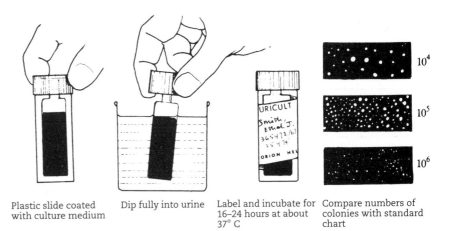

| Plastic slide coated with culture medium | Dip fully into urine | Label and incubate for 16–24 hours at about 37° C | Compare numbers of colonies with standard chart |

Fig. 2.6 Dip-slide method of estimating colony count.

bottle and incubated. After 12 h a glance at the chart supplied with the slides will tell whether there are over 10^5 colonies or not.

IMAGING THE URINARY TRACT

Plain abdominal radiograph ('scout film'; kidney, ureter and bladder, etc.)

Look at each film with four Ss in mind—side, skeleton, soft tissues and stones (Fig. 2.7).

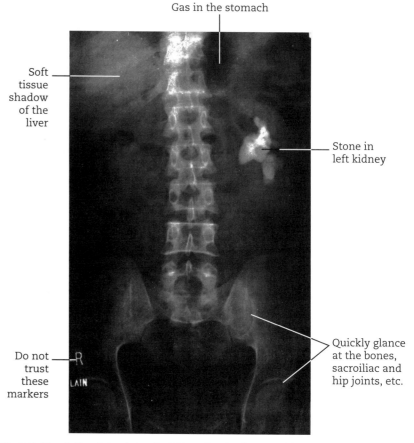

Gas in the stomach

Soft tissue shadow of the liver

Stone in left kidney

Do not trust these markers

Quickly glance at the bones, sacroiliac and hip joints, etc.

Fig. 2.7 Check the plain abdominal X-ray for the four Ss: side, skeleton, soft tissues and stones.

Side

Radiographers, being only human, may put the wrong letter on the film. Always check that the soft tissue shadow of the liver is on the right side and the gastric air bubble on the left.

Skeleton

Check the spine, ribs, hips and sacro-iliac joints for bony metastases, the evidence of ankylosing spondylitis, or loss of joint space in the hips which might have made the patient take analgesics and run the risk of analgesic nephropathy.

Soft tissues

In fat people the kidneys are surrounded by radiolucent fat which defines their outlines. A distended bladder or an enlarged uterus will fill the pelvis and displace the usual bowel gas shadows.

Stones

Any radio-opaque shadow in the line of the urinary tract might be a stone. If it seems to be in the kidney, it should move up and down with the kidney during respiration. 'Stones' in the pelvis often turn out to be calcified fibroids or phleboliths.

Ultrasound

Ultrasonography is cheap, painless and uses no dangerous radiation. Its principle is simple: remember how you could infuriate your schoolteacher by making the chalk squeak on the blackboard? You were making sound by applying force to the crystals of the chalk. The higher the pitch (frequency) the more annoying (penetrating) the squeak. The force applied to the crystal may be electric and at ultrasonic frequency will penetrate soft tissue but be reflected by bone and the interface between tissues of different density, e.g. renal calices and parenchyma, or the adenoma and capsule of the prostate (Fig. 2.8).

The returning echoes are received by a crystal which reverses the process and converts sound into an electrical impulse which is processed by a computer to give a cross-section through the body. Ultrasound images are more meaningful if you see them moving on a screen yourself, and much more if you perform the scan yourself.

Intravenous urogram or pyelogram

CONTRAST MEDIA

Its high atomic number makes iodine relatively opaque to X-rays. Free ionic iodine is toxic, but when joined to benzoic acid can form non-ionized organic salts

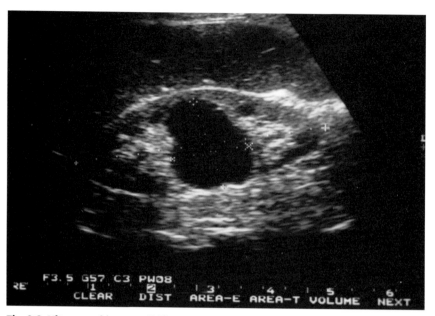

Fig. 2.8 Ultrasound image of kidney containing a cyst.

which can be given in large quantities, usually with safety but it does have its dangers.

Chemical irritation

To give a large enough quantity of contrast medium to provide a clear image requires a hypertonic solution. This irritates the vein causing pain to run up the arm and may cause a sterile chemical phlebitis which is easily mistaken for an infection.

When the bolus of hypertonic contrast medium reaches the systemic circulation it may cause nausea, flushing and sometimes vomiting. Neither of these side effects are serious but if the hypertonic solution extravasates into the soft tissue outside the vein it can cause a painful chemical inflammation and even skin necrosis.

Allergy

True allergy to contrast medium is even more serious. It can range from a trivial urticarial rash which will vanish with an antihistamine, to life-threatening oedema of the glottis, trachea and bronchi, with widespread vasodilatation, hypotension and cardiac arrest. Since the allergen is the whole iodobenzoate molecule, not free iodine, it is futile to perform skin tests with iodine. The reaction is not avoided by giving the first few millilitres of contrast slowly. The important precautions are always to enquire about even the most trivial previous reaction to contrast media, and to be ready for it in every case.

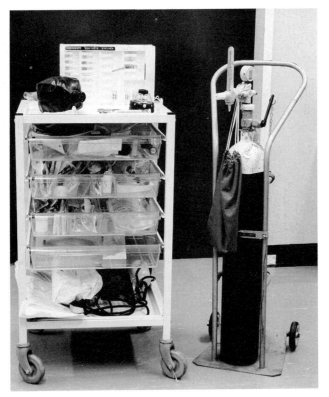

Fig. 2.9 Emergency kit to treat an allergic reaction to IVP contrast media.

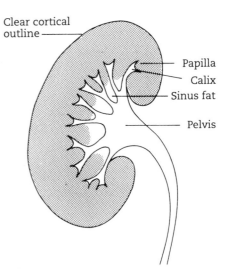

Fig. 2.10 Nephrogram phase of IVU.

Never start to give intravenous contrast medium without first making sure *for yourself* that all the essentials for treating an allergic reaction are to hand and within reach of the X-ray table: there must be adrenaline, hydrocortisone, oxygen, a face-mask, an airway, and a 'minitracheostomy' kit (Fig. 2.9). In every X-ray room there should be a 'panic button' that will summon the cardiac arrest team. Fatal reactions occur only in 1:200 000 intravenous urograms (IVUs), but millions of IVUs are done every year.

CONTRAST MEDIUM IN THE KIDNEY

It takes 15–20 s for the contrast medium to reach the kidney. A film taken in the first 30 s will catch the contrast as it lies in the glomeruli and proximal tubules where water is being reabsorbed, so this, the 'immediate' or 'nephrogram' film, gives an image of the renal parenchyma (Fig. 2.10). When it is particularly important to obtain a good picture of the renal outline, e.g. when scarring or a tumour are suspected, then tomograms taken during the nephrogram phase will eliminate unwanted shadows from gas in the bowel.

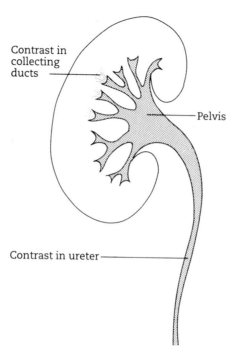

Contrast in collecting ducts

Pelvis

Contrast in ureter

Fig. 2.11 Pyelogram phase of IVU.

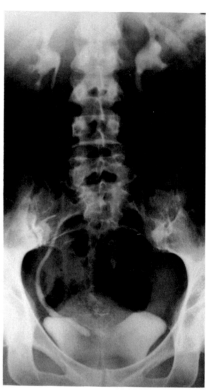

Fig. 2.12 The upper tracts and bladder are shown in the 20-min film of the IVU.

In obstruction the filtrate cannot escape down the tubule, and so the nephrogram is denser and lasts longer. With a stone blocking the ureter it is quite common to see the nephrogram persist for 24h or more.

In a normal patient the glomerular filtrate containing the contrast medium quickly reaches the calices and pelvis to give the pyelogram (Fig. 2.11). The calices can be filled out by compressing the abdomen with a tight band to squeeze the ureters for the first 10–15min, and a film taken just after releasing the band will then show the whole length of the ureter. Later films are taken to show the contrast in the bladder (Fig. 2.12).

The patient then empties the bladder, and if there is any question about the urethra, oblique films are taken during micturition to give a descending urethrogram. Afterwards a postmicturition film is taken which gives a rough idea of the volume of residual urine.

If one kidney is very small or scarred, most of the solute load has to be eliminated by the other one. In the small kidney the filtrate flows only slowly down the tubules, and in doing so becomes sufficiently concentrated to give a misleadingly clear image. Appearances are deceptive: never mistake a good image for good function.

PREPARATION FOR THE IVU

The obsolete practice still lingers of preparing patients for an IVU by depriving them of fluid for 6 h or longer. This may give a slight increase in the concentration of contrast in the filtrate, and perhaps a marginal improvement in the image, but in a normal patient given a normal amount of contrast the improvement does not justify the discomfort to the patient. Not only is the practice futile, it can be dangerous in diabetes, and in myeloma may lead to anuria from protein blocking the tubules.

Another obsolete practice was to purge the patient to get rid of gas shadows: again this can very seldom be justified.

To postpone an IVU merely because the patient 'is not prepared' should not be accepted as an excuse.

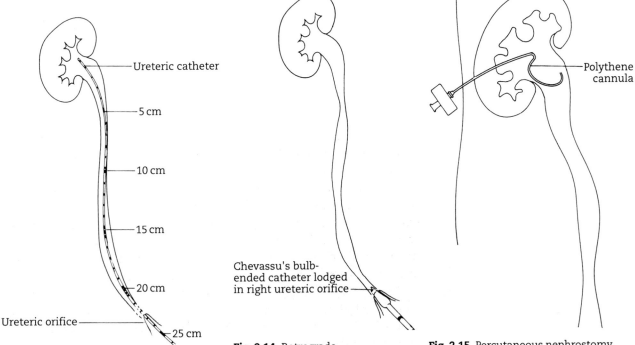

Fig. 2.13 Retrograde pyelogram with a ureteric catheter.

Fig. 2.14 Retrograde ureteropyelogram using a bulb-ended catheter.

Fig. 2.15 Percutaneous nephrostomy, to obtain descending or antegrade pyelogram.

Retrograde urogram

A fine ureteric catheter is passed up the ureteric orifice through a cystoscope and contrast medium is injected to outline the ureter and calices (Fig. 2.13). A similar image can be given by jamming a bulb-ended catheter in the ureteric orifice which will give an image of the whole length of the ureter (the ureterogram) (Fig. 2.14). Today these retrograde studies are performed under X-ray control.

Antegrade or descending urogram

A fine needle is passed into the renal pelvis under X-ray or ultrasound control. A flexible guide-wire is passed through the needle into the pelvis, the needle is withdrawn, and a cannula slipped over the guide-wire into the pelvis to perform a percutaneous nephrostomy (Fig. 2.15). This is the first step in a whole range of percutaneous operations on the kidney (see p. 82). Contrast medium injected through the cannula will delineate the renal pelvis and ureter. The pressure inside the cannula can be measured at the same time in the course of investigating obstruction (see p. 47).

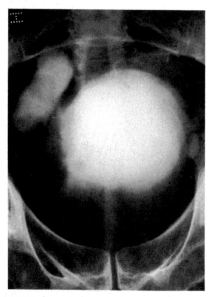

Fig. 2.16 Cystogram image at the end of the IVU, in this case showing a diverticulum on the right side of the bladder.

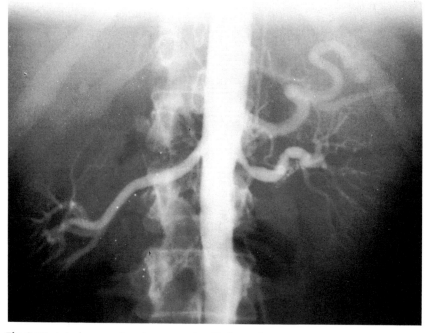

Fig. 2.17 Arteriogram showing stenosis of left renal artery.

Cystogram

For most purposes the image of the bladder given in the standard IVU will show diverticula or large tumours of the bladder (Fig. 2.16) but if the picture is not clear, or when it is necessary to rule out reflux from the bladder up the ureters, or in order to investigate incontinence, then the bladder is filled with contrast and screened while the patient passes urine. This is often combined with measurements of the pressure inside the bladder and the urine flow rate in a micturating cystometrogram (see p. 142).

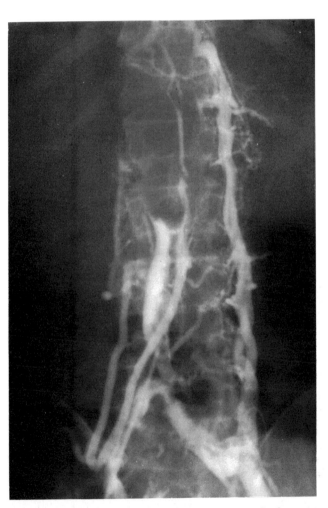

Fig. 2.18 Inferior vena cavogram showing tumour in the vena cava.

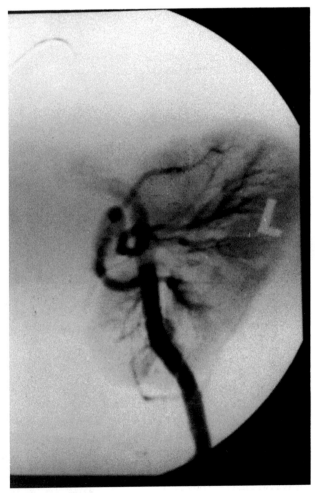

Fig. 2.19 Subtraction angiogram of a renal transplant in the left iliac fossa.

Urethrography

In investigating strictures and other disorders of the urethra an ascending ure-throgram is made by injecting contrast medium into the urethra with a small catheter (see p. 223).

Angiography

A flexible guide-wire is passed through a needle in the femoral artery over which a flexible cannula with a curved tip is slipped, and guided under X-ray control into the opening of the renal artery. Contrast is then injected into the renal artery or its branches to give an arteriogram (Fig. 2.17). This investigation is seldom needed but can be of value in the diagnosis of trauma, stenosis of the renal artery, and in some cases where the cause of haematuria is hard to discover. Similar studies are made when it is suspected that there may be extension of the tumour into the vena cava (cavography) (Fig. 2.18).

The image of smaller vessels in the angiogram can be improved if overlying shadows of bone and bowel gas are removed: this can be done with a computer (Fig. 2.19) to give a digital subtraction angiogram.

Computed tomography

In a conventional X-ray the image is a contact photograph of a phosphor which glows when bombarded with X-rays. Electronic sensors are far more sensitive

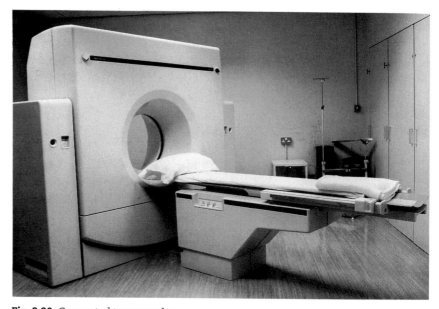

Fig. 2.20 Computed tomography.

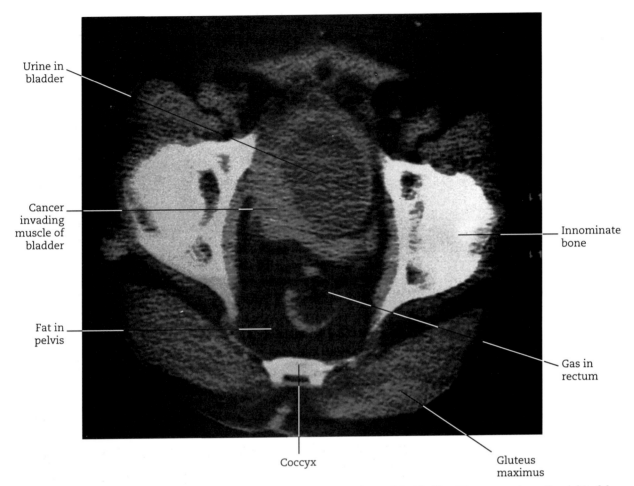

Urine in
bladder

Cancer
invading
muscle of
bladder

Innominate
bone

Fat in
pelvis

Gas in
rectum

Coccyx

Gluteus
maximus

Fig. 2.21 CT scan of a carcinoma of the bladder. The tumour is on the right of the bladder and has penetrated its wall.

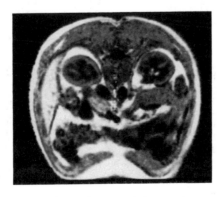

Fig. 2.22 MRI scan at the level of the kidneys. Courtesy of Dr G. Bidder.

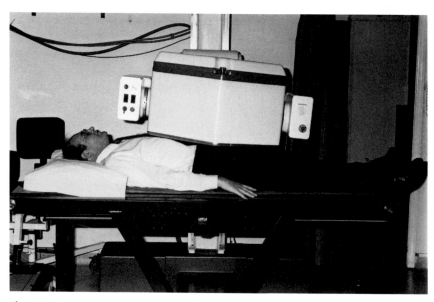

Fig. 2.23 Gamma camera. Courtesy of Dr C. A. Lewis.

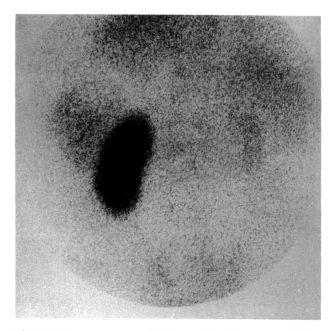

Fig. 2.24 Gamma camera DMSA scan showing a normal right kidney but almost no uptake on the left, due to severe scarring.

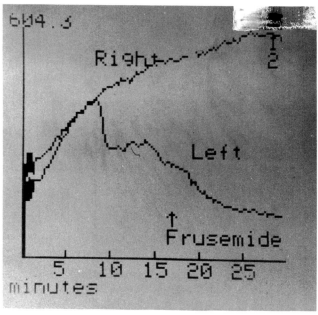

Fig. 2.25 DTPA renogram in a case of hydronephrosis showing hold up of contrast on the right side, in spite of frusemide.

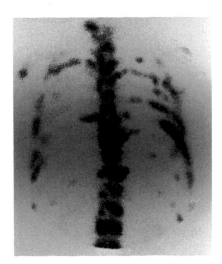

Fig. 2.26 Bone scan in a man with carcinoma of the prostate with widespread metastases.

than the phosphor in detecting small differences in radiodensity between one soft tissue and another. By mounting an array of these sensors in a hoop, through which the patient is passed in centimetre steps (Fig. 2.20), their signals can be processed by a computer to give an image of a transverse slice through the patient. Sir Godfrey Hounsfield, who invented the first chip computer and the computed tomography (CT) scanner, assigned an arbitrary scale of values (Hounsfield numbers) for the radiodensity of different tissues: −1000 for air, 0 for water, +1000 for bone (fat is about −100). Contrast medium can make the CT images even more precise (dynamic CT scanning) (Fig. 2.21).

Magnetic resonance imaging

Not content with the CT scanner, Hounsfield went on to devise an imaging system based on magnetism rather than X-rays. Atoms behave like gyroscopes whose axis can be tilted by a strong magnetic field. When the field is turned off the gyroscopes revert to their original position, and as they do so, give off a pulse of electromagnetic energy — magnetic resonance — which can be detected by another set of electronic sensors, mounted in a hoop and processed by computer to give an image (Fig. 2.22).

Isotope studies

Radionuclides are used to provide images and measure function. They are picked up and recorded by a gamma camera, a large flat sodium iodide crystal like a dinner plate, backed by an array of photomultiplier tubes, which amplify the small flashes of light emitted by the crystal as it is bombarded by the γ-rays from the isotopes (Fig. 2.23). These are either taken up by renal tubules, e.g. ^{99m}Tc dimercapto succinic acid (DMSA) (Fig. 2.24), filtered with the glomerular filtrate, e.g. ^{99m}Tc diethylene triamine pentacetic acid (DTPA) (Fig. 2.25), or taken up by bone in proportion to its blood supply, e.g. ^{99m}Tc methylene diphosphonate (MDP) (Fig. 2.26). A bone scan must always be interpreted with caution since many elderly men have arthritis and may have suffered fractured ribs from falls in the past.

FURTHER READING

Asscher AW, Sussman M, Waters WE, Davis RH, Chick S (1966) Urine as a medium for bacterial growth. *Lancet* **2**: 1037.

Kass EH (1956) Asymptomatic infections of the urinary tract. *Trans Ass Am Phys* **69**: 56.

Patel MD, Kricak H (1995) Current role of magnetic resonance imaging in urology. *Curr Op Urol* **5**: 67 (review).

Reidy JF (1988) Reactions to contrast media and steroid pretreatment. *Br Med J* **296**: 809.

Sarosdy MF, deVere White RW, Soloway MS et al. (1995) Results of a multicenter trial using the BTA test to monitor for and diagnose recurrent bladder cancer. *J Urol* **154**: 379.

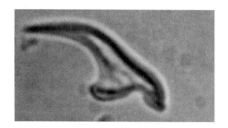

The Kidney: Structure and Function

Surgical relations of the kidney

The kidneys are well protected, tucked in on either side of the spine. In front is the liver: behind there is the lung, constantly moving up and down. In anatomical terms the posterior relations of the kidney are the 12th rib, diaphragm, pleura and lung (Fig. 3.1), and below them the quadratus lumborum and psoas muscles. The ilioinguinal and hypogastric nerves cross the quadratus lumborum muscle and so are always injured to some extent in operating on the kidney. Since the kidney moves up and down in respiration, at any one time it may be anywhere between the level of the 2nd and 3rd transverse processes of the lumbar vertebrae.

LEFT KIDNEY

The tail of the pancreas and the spleen lie in front of the left kidney; either of these are easily injured at operation. The duodenojejunal flexure and descending colon also lie just in front of the left kidney, so indigestion or bowel distension is common when there is inflammation or obstruction of the kidney, and cancer of the kidney easily invades the adjacent bowel (Figs 3.2, 3.3).

RIGHT KIDNEY

In front of the right kidney are the ascending colon, the second part of the duodenum and the common bile duct: it is not surprising that 'indigestion' so often accompanies disorders of the right kidney (Figs 3.4, 3.5).

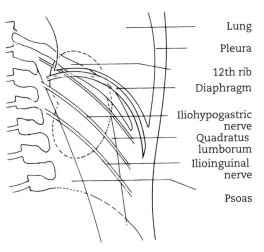

Lung
Pleura
12th rib
Diaphragm
Iliohypogastric
nerve
Quadratus
lumborum
Ilioinguinal
nerve
Psoas

Fig. 3.1 Posterior anatomical relations of the kidney.

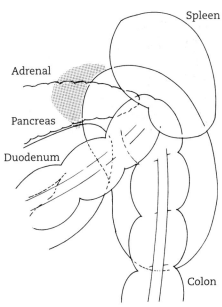

Spleen
Adrenal
Pancreas
Duodenum
Colon

Fig. 3.2 Anatomical relations of the left kidney.

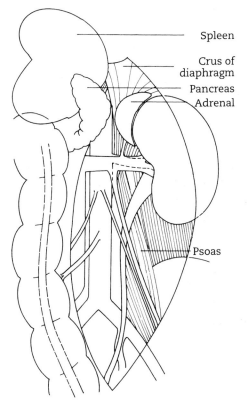

Spleen
Crus of diaphragm
Pancreas
Adrenal
Psoas

Fig. 3.3 Left kidney and surrounding structures displayed at operation by reflecting the colon, spleen and tail of pancreas medially.

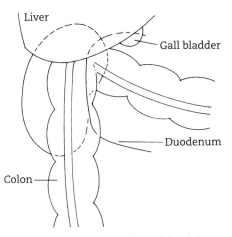

Liver
Gall bladder
Duodenum
Colon

Fig. 3.4 Anatomical relations of the right kidney.

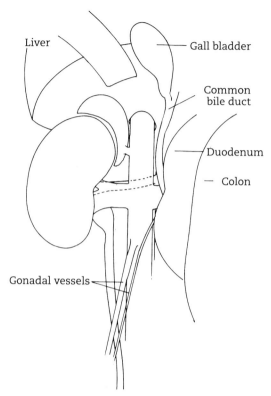

Fig. 3.5 Right kidney and surrounding structures displayed at operation by reflecting the colon and duodenum medially.

Surgical approaches to the kidney

POSTERIOR

Percutaneous nephrostomy

When a needle is passed into the renal pelvis (see p. 20) it must pass through skin, latissimum dorsi, quadratus lumborum, perirenal fat and renal parenchyma to reach the renal pelvis. It is easy to understand how by mischance the needle may pierce the pleura, liver, duodenum or colon.

Twelfth rib approach

Most open operations on the kidney are performed through an incision along the bed of the 12th rib which intends to avoid opening the pleura (but often does). The 11th and 12th subcostal nerves as well as the ilioinguinal and hypogastric nerves are always stretched and sometimes cut. Postoperative pain is often quite severe (Fig. 3.6).

Vertical lumbotomy
A vertical incision along the lateral border of sacrospinalis may free the attachments of the abdominal muscles, giving limited access to the kidney but avoiding much of the pain of the 12th rib approach (Fig. 3.7).

Thoracoabdominal incision
For very large cancers safety demands perfect exposure. The incision is carried through the bed of the 10th rib, across the pleura and into the abdomen. The lung and liver are retracted. The improved access to the inferior vena cava and aorta allows the surgeon to avoid and control bleeding.

ANTERIOR APPROACHES

Minimal access surgery

Extraperitoneal
Through a cannula introduced into the perirenal fat, a balloon is passed and blown up to separate the peritoneum, duodenum and colon from the kidney. It is kept blown up long enough for bleeding to stop, and then deflated, leaving an empty

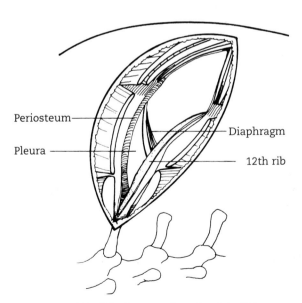

Fig. 3.6 Twelfth rib bed approach to the right kidney.

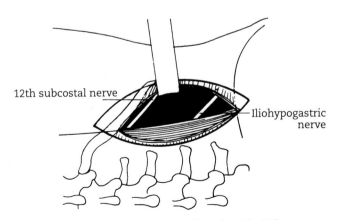

Fig. 3.7 Vertical lumbotomy approach to the right kidney.

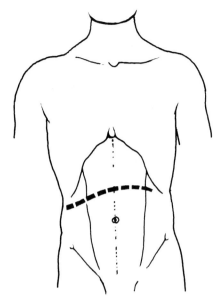

Fig. 3.8 Anterior transabdominal approach to right kidney through a transverse incision.

space into which laparoscopic instruments may be introduced to carry out various operations on the kidney.

Transperitoneal
Carbon dioxide is introduced into the peritoneal cavity with a small cannula and then a number of 'ports' are made through which large cannulae are pushed into the gas-filled space. Through these other instruments are passed to reflect the colon and duodenum off the front of the kidney and allow the planned operation to take place.

Conventional open surgery
With a large cancer of the kidney safety demands perfect exposure to control the renal artery and vein. The choice of either a transverse or midline incision is determined by the build of the patient (Figs 3.8, 3.9). The colon and duodenum are reflected medially to give safe access to the renal vessels (Figs 3.10, 3.11).

COMPLICATIONS AFTER RENAL SURGERY
The surgical relations of the kidney explain most of the common postoperative complications.

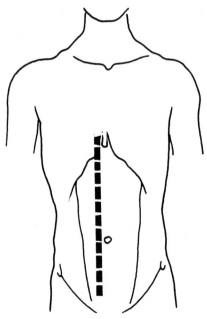

Fig. 3.9 Transabdominal approach through vertical incision in a long thin patient.

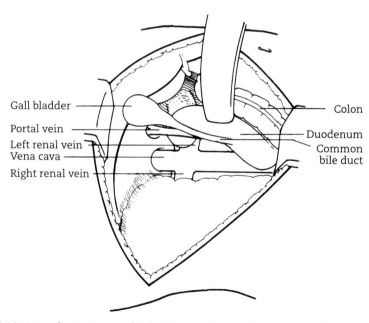

Fig. 3.10 Operative exposure of right kidney: colon and duodenum reflected.

Gall bladder
Portal vein
Left renal vein
Vena cava
Right renal vein
Colon
Duodenum
Common bile duct

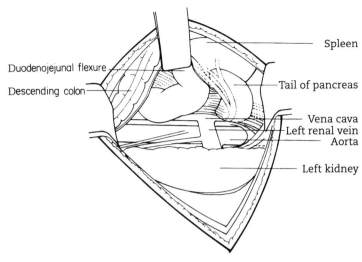

Fig. 3.11 Operative exposure of left kidney: spleen, colon and duodenum reflected.

Pain

There is always postoperative pain on breathing and coughing. Postoperative pain can inhibit coughing and lead to atelectasis and infection in the empty lung segments. This is more common when the pleura has been opened or if part of the rib has had to be removed.

Pneumothorax

This may require aspiration or underwater drainage.

Ileus

Oedema or haematoma behind the bowel may lead to a period of abdominal distension and paralytic ileus.

STRUCTURE OF THE KIDNEY

Renal pyramid

The basic unit of the mammalian kidney is the pyramid. In porpoises the pyramids remain separate so that the kidney looks like a bunch of grapes. In most other mammals, including humans, the porpoise arrangement is seen only in the fetus; in the adult, the dozen pyramids are squeezed together (Fig. 3.12). Each pyramid is

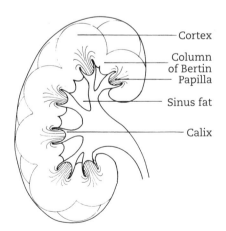

Fig. 3.12 The kidney is formed of a collection of pyramids squeezed together: where they merge they form the columns of Bertin.

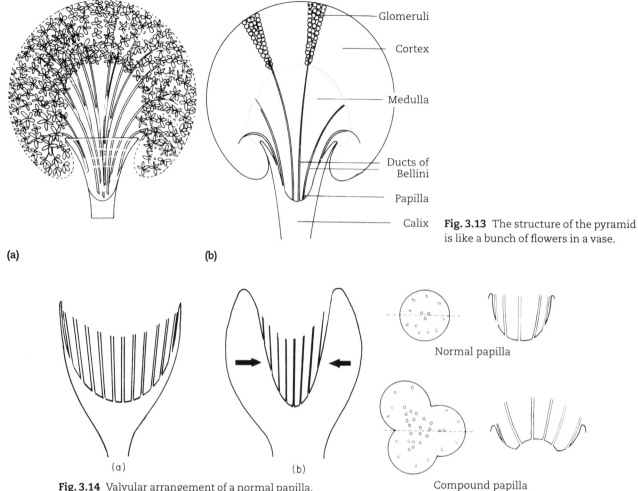

(a)   (b)

Fig. 3.13 The structure of the pyramid is like a bunch of flowers in a vase.

(a)   (b)

Fig. 3.14 Valvular arrangement of a normal papilla.

Normal papilla

Compound papilla

Fig. 3.15 Normal (above) and compound papillae.

like a bunch of flowers in a vase (Fig. 3.13), the blooms are the glomeruli, the stems the collecting ducts and the whole bunch, the papilla, sits in a vase, the calix.

RENAL PAPILLA

The collecting ducts open onto the papilla obliquely so that when pressure rises in the calix the ducts are closed (Fig. 3.14). Children may be born with papillae that are fused together—compound papillae. This makes the valve mechanism ineffective so if there is obstruction or reflux urine is forced into the renal parenchyma causing inflammation and scarring (see p. 59) (Fig. 3.15).

The collecting ducts gather the glomerular filtrate from the convoluted tubules of each nephron. The nephrons are arranged like corn on the cob (Fig. 3.16). Each nephron has two parts: a filter, the glomerulus, and a processing plant, the renal tubules.

GLOMERULUS

Each glomerulus is made of an arteriole, coiled like a ball of wool, which is invaginated into a hollow balloon — Bowman's capsule — whose stem drains into the proximal tubule (Fig. 3.17). The glomerular arteriole is very permeable, with an endothelium specially dimpled to increase its porosity. Its basement membrane is supported like filter paper on a grid formed by the foot-processes of the epithelial cells of Bowman's capsule, which interlock like a zip-fastener

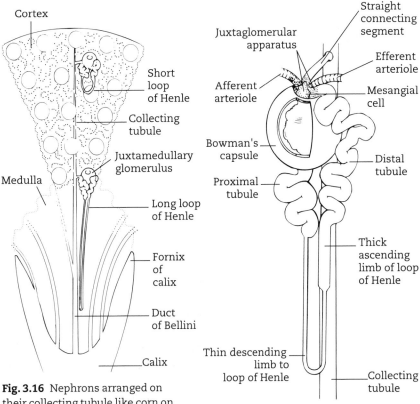

Fig. 3.16 Nephrons arranged on their collecting tubule like corn on the cob.

Fig. 3.17 A nephron.

(Fig. 3.18). The spaces between the zip are called 'slit-pores' and their size can be measured using peroxidases of known molecular mass: these measurements show that those of molecular mass less than 40 000 can slip through: those above 160 000 get stuck.

Filtration is not merely a matter of the size of the molecule. The proteins of the basement membrane are negatively charged and repel negatively charged molecules, e.g. albumen, but allow positively charged molecules of similar size to pass through.

The pressure inside the glomerular arteriole is about 60 mmHg. The plasma oncotic pressure is about 25 mmHg, so that there is a filtration pressure of about 35 mmHg. The pressure inside Bowman's capsule is about 10 mmHg.

The arterioles of the glomeruli are 50 times more permeable than those of arterioles elsewhere, e.g. muscle, and they allow enormous volumes of fluid to leak out. The whole plasma water is filtered every 30 min and the entire body water processed four times a day. The first task of the tubules is to recapture this huge amount of water.

Tests of glomerular function

For most purposes the plasma creatinine is an adequate guide to glomerular func-

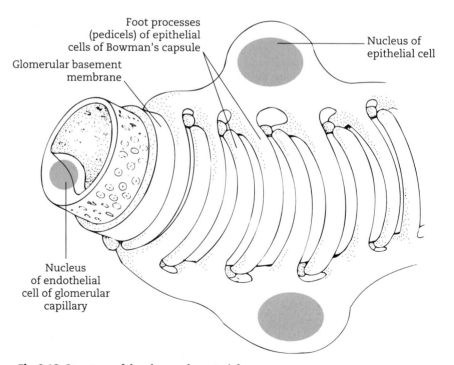

Fig. 3.18 Structure of the glomerular arteriole.

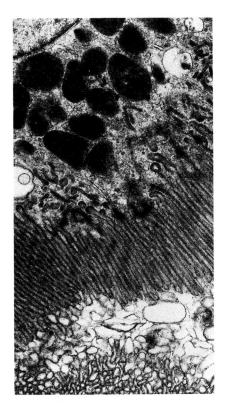

Fig. 3.19 Electron photomicrograph showing the brush border of the proximal renal tubule. Courtesy of Dr Jo Martin.

tion. Occasionally a more precise measure is needed. The classical test used to be the creatinine clearance. This required an exactly timed collection of urine, which was difficult in a busy hospital ward. The plasma creatinine was then measured at some convenient time. Clearance was given by the formula UV/P where U = urine creatinine mg/100 ml, V = urine volume in ml/min, and P = plasma creatinine mg/100 ml. The answer was expressed in ml/min. The main source of error was the timed collection of urine and for this reason creatinine clearance has been superseded by diethylene triamine pentacetic acid (DTPA) clearance (see p. 25). ^{99m}Tc-labelled DTPA is given and the rate of disappearance from the kidney or forearm measured with a gamma camera.

RENAL TUBULES

Proximal tubule

About 75% of the excess water is reabsorbed in the proximal tubule, which is lined with active cells whose surface area is enormously increased by their brush border of microvilli (Fig. 3.19). These metabolically busy cells also recover glucose, phosphate and amino acids from the glomerular filtrate.

Loop of Henle

The filtrate now passes through the loops of Henle. Most of these are quite short, but those in the inner part of the pyramid dip down like hairpins into the papilla, where they run alongside collecting tubules. The cells of the loops of Henle are thin, and allow osmosis to withdraw salt and water from the glomerular filtrate into the concentrated tissue of the papilla. So-called 'loop diuretics', e.g. frusemide, inhibit Cl^- transport, reduce hypertonicity in the papilla, and allow more water to escape along with potassium. This effect is further potentiated by spironolactone (see p. 107).

Distal tubule

The filtrate now rises up into the distal convoluted tubule whose cells are thick and metabolically active but have no brush border. They exchange Na^+ for K^+ and H^+ ions to regulate the acid–base balance of the body. Disease of the distal convoluted tubules prevents the urine from forming an acid urine, the so-called renal tubular acidosis.

Collecting tubules

Leaving the distal convoluted tubule the filtrate enters the collecting tubule, and once more runs the gauntlet of the hypertonic papilla. Here the last fine tuning of the reabsorption of water takes place under the control of the pituitary antidiuretic hormone.

Tests of tubular function

DMSA
The rate of uptake of ^{99m}Tc DMSA is recorded by a gamma camera (see p. 25). This is the usual test of renal tubular function. Only occasionally is it necessary to use the classical tests.

Acid load
After collecting two 1-h specimens of urine over 2 h, the patient is given NH_4Cl in gelatin-coated capsules (0.1 g/kg body weight) in a litre of water over 1 h. Three hours later a third 1-h specimen of urine is collected. Healthy distal tubules can handle this by secreting urine with a pH over 5.3, a titratable acidity over 25 mmol/min and over 35 mmol/min of ammonium. In practice the NH_4Cl often makes patients vomit and the test is void.

Urine concentration test
The patient may be deprived of water, or given desmopressin, an analogue of pituitary antidiuretic hormone (40 μg/kg for adults, 20 μg/kg for children) and the specific gravity of the urine is measured over the next 6 h. The test must never be attempted in patients with renal failure.

BLOOD SUPPLY OF THE KIDNEY
Every operation on the kidney reminds the surgeon of its rich blood supply: between them the kidneys receive one-fifth of the entire cardiac output, and the first step in any operation is to get control of the renal artery. Usually there is one renal artery on each side, each with five segmental branches arranged like the digits of the hand (Fig. 3.20). Each segmental branch supplies its own geographical zone of the parenchyma and there is no anastomosis between them (Fig. 3.21).

The zones supplied by the segmental arteries do not match the arrangement of pyramids and calices. In open operations any incision into the renal parenchyma is made between the main segmental arteries, which can be located with a Doppler probe (Fig. 3.22).

Each segmental artery divides into smaller arcuate arteries which run in the boundary between cortex and medulla, giving off branches which run up and down parallel with the collecting tubules, as well as giving an afferent artery to each glomerulus (Fig. 3.23).

The afferent artery enters the glomerulus near the junction of the loop of Henle with the distal convoluted tubule: the juxtaglomerular apparatus is located here; its cells contain dark granules of the precursor of renin. The juxtaglomerular apparatus monitors the pressure in the afferent arteriole (see p. 104).

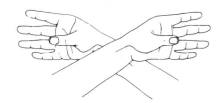

Fig. 3.20 Arrangement of the branches of the renal arteries.

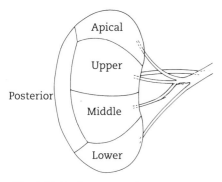

Fig. 3.21 Each segmental artery supplies its own geographical territory.

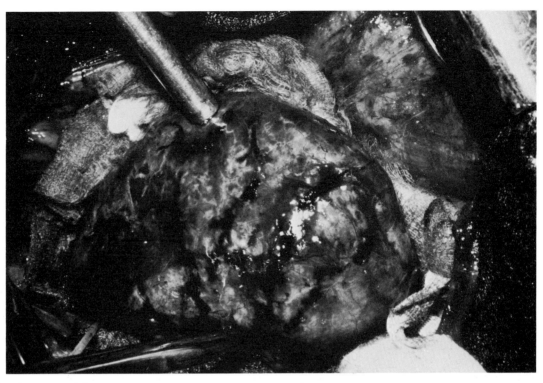

Fig. 3.22 At operation the segmental arteries can be located with a Doppler probe so that an incision into the parenchyma can avoid them.

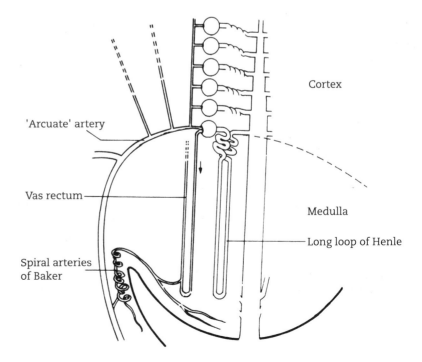

'Arcuate' artery

Vas rectum

Spiral arteries
of Baker

Cortex

Medulla

Long loop of Henle

Fig. 3.23 The blood supply of the renal papilla.

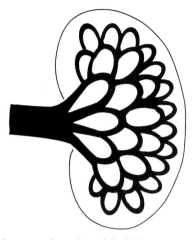

Fig. 3.24 The veins of the kidney communicate with each other.

RENAL VEINS

Unlike the neat territories supplied by the branches of the renal arteries, the veins all communicate freely with each other (Fig. 3.24) so several veins can be ligated without infarcting the kidney. The main left renal vein often splits into two, one part running in front of the aorta, the other behind, posing a trap for the surgeon who is unaware of this anomaly. The left renal vein is about 5 cm long, the right is close to the inferior vena cava, another reason why the left kidney is preferred in live-donor transplantation.

THE COLLECTING SYSTEM

The thin cubical epithelium of the papilla is perforated with the collecting ducts (of Bellini) but the rest of the pelvis and calix is lined by urothelium like that of the bladder and ureters. The urothelium is surrounded by a wall of smooth muscle

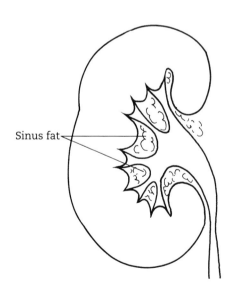

Sinus fat

Fig. 3.26 The calices are surrounded by sinus fat which is fluid at body temperature and allows them to move freely.

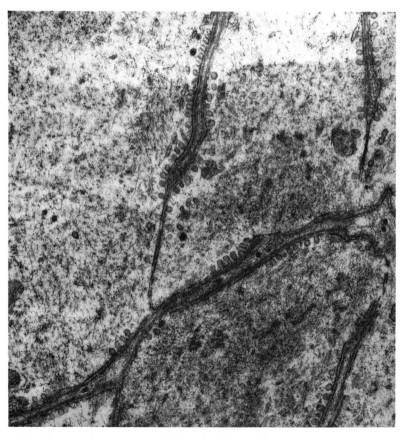

Fig. 3.25 Electron photomicrograph showing jigsaw connections between cells (nexuses). Courtesy of Mr R.G. Notley.

cells linked by jigsaw connections, nexuses, which transmit the wave of contraction from one muscle cell to another without the need for any nerve supply, so a transplanted kidney continues to pump out urine perfectly well (Fig. 3.25).

The calices are separated from the renal parenchyma by a packing of sinus fat which is fluid at body temperature, and allows them to contract freely (Fig. 3.26).

FURTHER READING

Blandy JP, Fowler CG (1996) Kidney and ureter—anatomy and physiology. In: Blandy JP (ed.) *Urology*, 2nd edn. Oxford, Blackwell Science, pp. 39–63.

Brown SCW, O'Reilly PH (1995) Glomerular filtration rate measurement a neglected test in urological practice. *Br J Urol* **75**: 296.

Dixon JS, Gosling JA (1990) Fundamentals of renal anatomy. In: Chisholm GD, Fair WR (eds) *Scientific Foundations of Urology*, 3rd edn. Oxford, Heinemann, pp. 1–10.

Graves FT (1971) *The Arterial Anatomy of the Kidney: the Basis of Surgical Technique*. Bristol, John Wright.

Jamison RL, Gehrig JJ (1992) Urinary concentration and dilution: physiology. In: Windhager EE (ed.) *Handbook of Physiology 9*, vol 1 *Renal Physiology*. Oxford, Oxford University Press, pp. 639–57.

Marshall FF (1978) Embryology of the lower genitourinary tract. *Urol Clin N Am* **5**: 3.

Mattiessen TB, Rittig S, Norgaard JP, Pedersen EB, Djurhuus JC (1996) Nocturnal polyuria and natriuresis in male patients with nocturia and lower urinary tract symptoms. *J Urol* **156**: 1291.

Nakamura S, Koayashi Y, Tozuka K, Tokue A, Kimura A, Hamada C (1996) Circadian changes in urine volume and frequency in elderly men. *J Urol* **156**: 1275.

Reidy JF (1988) Reactions to contrast media and steroid pretreatment. *Br Med J* **296**: 809.

Smith HW (1953) *From Fish to Philosopher*. Boston, Little, Brown.

Stephenson JL (1992) Urinary concentration and dilution. In: Windhager EE (ed.) *Handbook of Physiology 9*, vol. 1 *Renal Physiology*. Oxford, Oxford University Press, pp. 1219–79.

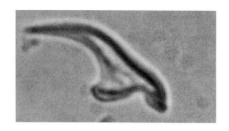

The Kidney: Congenital Disorders

Primitive vertebrates were constructed like a railway train: each identical somite had a pair of nephrons which allowed fluid from the coelom to leak out into the surrounding sea. Later on these nephrons came to be arranged into three groups: the most cranial of these, the pronephros, is today only an evolutionary curiosity, found in a few fish embryos, but of no conceivable relevance to humans. The second set, the mesonephros, corresponds to the functioning kidney of present day fish and frogs whose mesonephric or Wolffian duct empties urine into the cloaca.

In humans the mesonephros has disappeared. Our kidneys are derived from a third, more caudal set of nephrons — the metanephros — which drains into a branch of the caudal end of the mesonephric duct—the ureter (Fig. 4.1).

The mesonephric duct persists in males as the vas deferens. If the mesonephric duct fails to develop, then there is neither ureter, kidney nor vas deferens on that side—renal agenesis (Fig. 4.2).

A second pair of ducts develops parallel to the mesonephric ducts: these are the paramesonephric or Müllerian ducts. In females they form the fallopian tubes, which fuse in the midline to form the uterus. In males they persist as a pit on the verumontanum in the prostatic urethra—the utriculus masculinus—as well as a tiny cyst attached to the upper pole of the testis which is only of interest because it sometimes twists on its stalk and mimics torsion of the testicle (see p. 260).

DUPLEX KIDNEY AND URETER

After budding out from the lower end of the mesonephric duct, the ureter usually begins to branch when it gets near the metanephros but sometimes it divides earlier and may produce a complete double system of renal pelvis and calices—ren

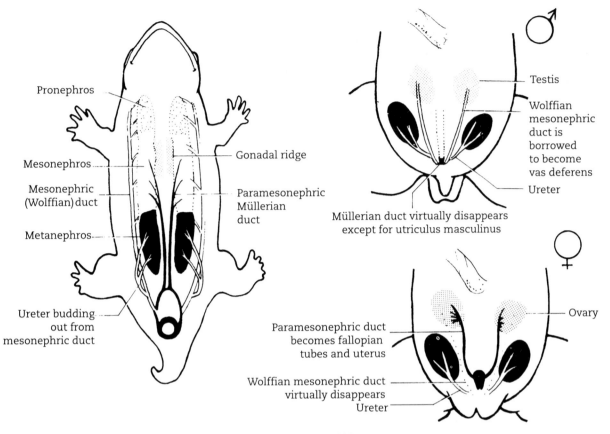

Fig. 4.1 Embryology of the kidney.

duplex. The overlying renal parenchyma is never completely separated but a distinct 'waist' marks the distinction between the two halves, as does a prominent bulge in the parenchyma, which is sometimes mistaken for a carcinoma in X-rays (Fig. 4.3).

The upper half kidney has two main calices, the lower half has three and makes more urine. Urine may be squirted from the lower half up into the upper half, causing distension and pain—yo-yo reflux (Fig. 4.4).

While the ureters are budding out towards the metanephros (Fig. 4.5) a shutter of tissue, the urogenital septum, grows down to separate the bladder in front from the rectum behind. The septum carries with it the mesonephric duct and the ureteric buds which are bent into a loop. The lower part of the mesonephric duct is absorbed into the trigone of the future bladder (Fig. 4.6). The upper part of the mesonephric duct—taken over as the vas deferens in the male—swings down with the testis into the scrotum (Fig. 4.7).

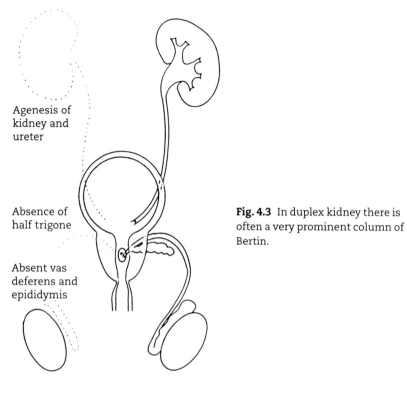

Agenesis of kidney and ureter

Absence of half trigone

Absent vas deferens and epididymis

Fig. 4.2 Renal agenesis.

Fig. 4.3 In duplex kidney there is often a very prominent column of Bertin.

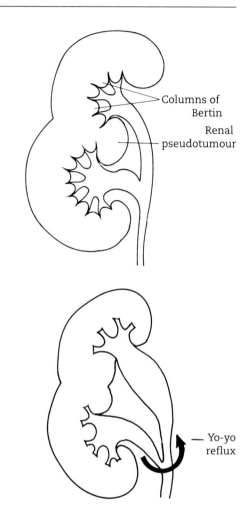

Columns of Bertin

Renal pseudotumour

Yo-yo reflux

Fig. 4.4 Yo-yo reflux.

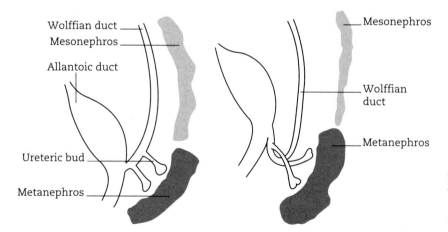

Wolffian duct
Mesonephros
Allantoic duct

Ureteric bud

Metanephros

Mesonephros

Wolffian duct

Metanephros

Fig. 4.5 Two ureteric buds from the Wolffian duct reach the metanephros, and then the Wolffian duct is bent round.

A duplex kidney is nearly always innocent and symptomless, but it can be associated with three conditions that cause trouble: ectopic ureter, reflux and ureterocele.

1 Ectopic ureter. If the ureter draining the upper half kidney opens into the vagina, caudal to the sphincter, it gives rise to continual incontinence (Fig. 4.8).

2 Reflux. Because the ureter from the lower half kidney has a relatively short course through the wall of the bladder it has a less efficient valve, and urine may reflux from the bladder up to the kidney (Fig. 4.9).

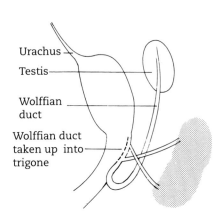

Urachus

Testis

Wolffian duct

Wolffian duct taken up into trigone

Fig. 4.6 The lower end of the Wolffian duct is incorporated into the bladder.

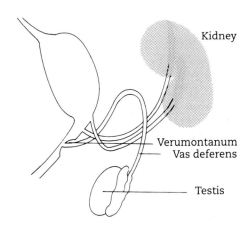

Kidney

Verumontanum
Vas deferens

Testis

Fig. 4.7 The Wolffian duct becomes the vas deferens.

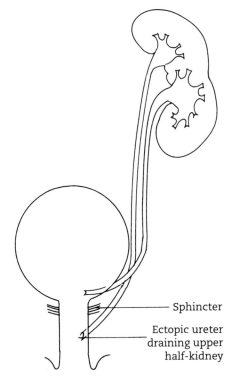

Sphincter

Ectopic ureter draining upper half-kidney

Fig. 4.8 If the ureter from the upper half kidney opens below the sphincter in a girl there is continual incontinence.

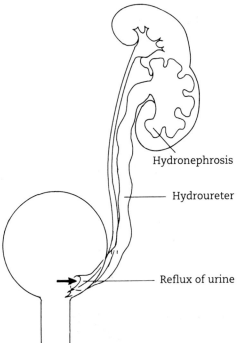

Hydronephrosis

Hydroureter

Reflux of urine

Fig. 4.9 Reflux up the lower ureter into the upper half kidney.

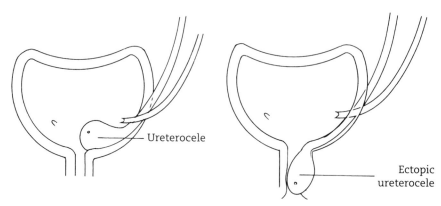

Fig. 4.10 A ureterocele may prolapse into the urethra.

3   Ureterocele. If the lower end of the mesonephric duct is incompletely absorbed into the trigone it may form a balloon just where the ureter enters the trigone—ureterocele. This may be found with a normal single ureter, but is more often seen at the lower of two ureteric orifices in complete duplex. Very occasionally a ureterocele may prolapse out of the urethra as a translucent 'cyst' causing painful acute retention of urine (Fig. 4.10).

ERRORS OF POSITION OF THE KIDNEY

ROTATED KIDNEY

A kidney often faces forwards rather than medially. Its outline is then an ellipse and some of its calices point medially (Fig. 4.11). Such a 'rotated kidney' is entirely harmless.

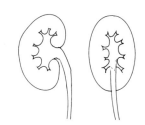

Fig. 4.11 Rotated kidney.

HORSESHOE KIDNEY

Here not only are both kidneys rotated, but their lower poles are joined in the shape of a horseshoe (Fig. 4.12). This happens if the two metanephroi get fused together in the fetal pelvis: the reason for this is unknown. As the fetus grows, the joined kidneys are held up by the inferior or superior mesenteric arteries. In operations for aortic aneurysm, the isthmus joining the two kidneys may have to be divided, but otherwise it should be left alone.

Reflux, ureterocele and hydronephrosis are often found in association with a horseshoe kidney, and should be dealt with in the usual way, without meddling with the isthmus.

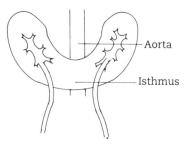

Fig. 4.12 Horseshoe kidney.

CROSSED RENAL ECTOPIA

Instead of being united in the midline like a horseshoe, the two kidneys may fuse

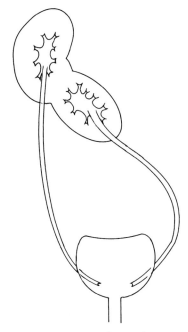

together on one side. Their ureters always run along their proper side. As with horseshoe kidney, there is often some other congenital anomaly such as reflux or obstruction (Fig. 4.13).

PELVIC KIDNEY

Here the metanephros remains in the pelvis. One might expect it would get in the way of the baby during childbirth, but it hardly ever does. A pelvic kidney is usually detected by chance, and seldom needs any treatment unless associated with some other condition such as hydronephrosis. But there is one unexpected and important hazard: at laparotomy for abdominal pain an unwary surgeon comes across an unusual 'tumour' and goes ahead to remove it. These pelvic kidneys have their segmental arteries arising separately from the aorta, common and internal iliac arteries which can cause confusion and bleeding if the condition is not recognized (Fig. 4.14).

THORACIC KIDNEY

This is not so much an error of development of the kidney as of the diaphragm, where one kidney is carried up into the chest along with other viscera. Such a 'thoracic' kidney is found by chance in a chest radiograph or an intravenous urogram (IVU). The kidney is not really in the thorax: a thin layer of diaphragm and pleura always separate the two compartments. The kidney itself needs no treatment (Fig. 4.15).

Fig. 4.13 Crossed renal ectopia.

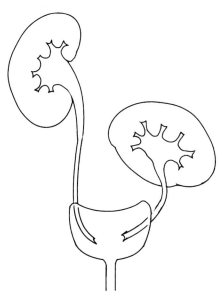

Fig. 4.14 Pelvic kidney.

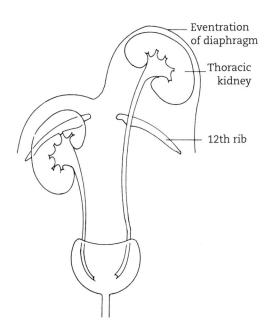

Eventration of diaphragm

Thoracic kidney

12th rib

Fig. 4.15 Thoracic kidney.

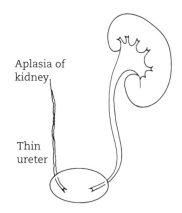

Aplasia of kidney

Thin ureter

Fig. 4.16 Aplasia.

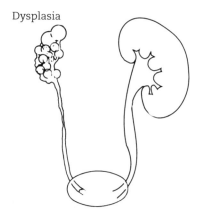

Dysplasia

Fig. 4.17 Dysplasia.

ERRORS OF DEVELOPMENT OF THE KIDNEY

In agenesis the entire mesonephric duct fails to develop so there is an absence of ureter, trigone, kidney and (in boys) vas deferens (see Fig. 4.2). Although the mesonephric duct develops properly, the ureteric bud may not. Because the metanephros cannot develop properly without the ureter, the metanephros may not differentiate at all — aplasia (Fig. 4.16) — or it may develop poorly, with odd-looking tissue including little cysts and lumps of cartilage — dysplasia (Fig. 4.17). Hypoplasia is a term to avoid: it implies that the kidney is small but otherwise normal: which is never the case.

CYSTIC DISORDERS OF THE KIDNEY

Medullary sponge kidney

Here the collecting ducts are grossly dilated (Fig. 4.18). Part or all of one or both kidneys may be affected, and the medulla becomes swollen and honeycombed with cysts giving the appearance of a sponge. The radiographic appearance is characteristic (Fig. 4.19). Infection in the dilated tubules is soon followed by the development of numerous small stones which give repeated attacks of ureteric colic. With extracorporeal lithotripsy the larger stones can be broken up and allowed to pass before they give rise to serious trouble, but repeated attacks of infection and scarring ultimately leads to renal failure.

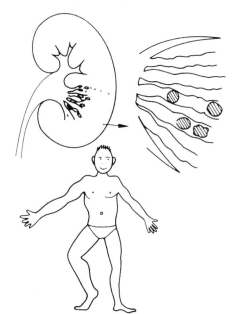

Fig. 4.18 Medullary sponge kidney: dilated collecting tubules and unilateral hemihypertrophy of the body.

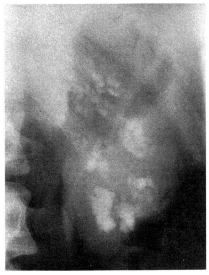

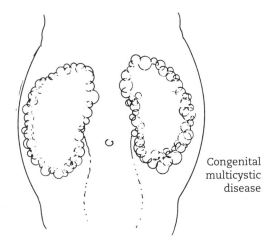

Congenital multicystic disease

Fig. 4.20 Congenital multicystic kidney.

Fig. 4.19 X-ray of medullary sponge kidney showing multiple calculi in dilated collecting ducts.

Obstruction cysts

CONGENITAL OBSTRUCTION OF THE URETER

The ureter may become narrowed in fetal life for causes as yet unknown. The kidney continues to make urine, and the nephrons become distended, converting the kidney into a so-called congenital multicystic kidney (Fig. 4.20). If the condition is bilateral the fetus forms no urine, so there is no amniotic fluid, and the baby's face is characteristically flattened — Potter's facies (Fig. 4.21). There are usually several other congenital anomalies of the cardiovascular and other systems and the condition is incompatible with life.

A minor version of this imperfect development of the ureter is seen where there is a tiny, thin ureter, above which a small kidney is found, largely converted into small cysts—cystic dysplasia.

A single calix may become obstructed, and the pyramid draining into it becomes converted into a hollow bag—caliceal cyst. These seem to be congenital, and are only found if infection or stones develop in the cyst (Fig. 4.22).

ACQUIRED OBSTRUCTION

Rather similar cysts occur as a consequence of the scarring and contraction which takes place in the later stages of pyelonephritis. The obstructed nephrons occasionally become grossly distended with protein (Fig. 4.23). This kind of cyst is

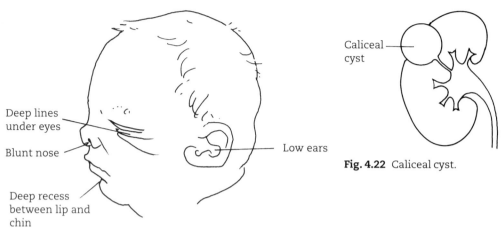

Deep lines under eyes

Blunt nose

Deep recess between lip and chin

Low ears

Fig. 4.21 Potter's facies.

Caliceal cyst

Fig. 4.22 Caliceal cyst.

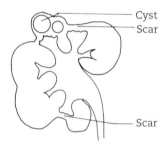

Cyst

Scar

Scar

Fig. 4.23 Obstructed cysts in pyelonephritic scarring.

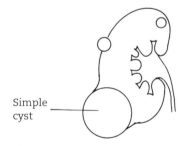

Simple cyst

Fig. 4.24 Simple cysts of the kidney.

being seen more often as more patients with end-stage renal failure now survive for many years on dialysis.

Diverticula of the collecting tubules

The usual type of renal cysts arise as diverticula from the collecting tubules of the kidney. One or more of these simple cysts occur in middle age in almost every otherwise normal kidney. They are often picked up by accident in an ultrasound scan (Fig. 4.24) and nothing needs to be done about them (Fig. 4.25). Occasionally these simple cysts may grow big enough to obstruct a calix and cause pain, especially if they arise from the medulla (parapelvic cysts). They can easily be emptied by fine-needle aspiration, and if they fill up again, can be uncapped at an open or percutaneous procedure. Very rarely the fluid inside a cyst becomes infected and requires drainage.

Polycystic disease

A bizarre exaggeration of this process is seen in polycystic disease. There are two main forms of this condition: childhood and adult.

Childhood polycystic disease (Fig. 4.26)

This type of polycystic disease is inherited as a Mendelian recessive characteristic and occurs at four different ages.

1   Fetal. Ultrasound reveals that both kidneys have been converted into giant sponges. It is not compatible with survival.

2   Neonatal. A similar condition is discovered in the neonate, who may survive for up to a year, unless a transplant can be found.

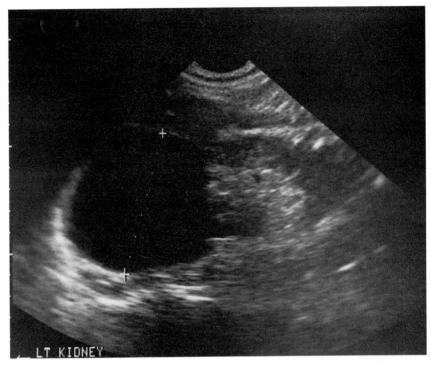

Fig. 4.25 Ultrasound showing a simple cyst. Courtesy of Dr W. Hately.

3 Infantile. Between 3 and 6 months these children are found to have uraemia and enlarged kidneys; there is also an associated fibrosis of the portal system.
4 Juvenile. This is discovered in later childhood, and is also associated with hepatic fibrosis.

Adult polycystic disease (Fig. 4.27)

This is inherited by an autosomal dominant gene on chromosome 16. It may appear in children, but is usually diagnosed in adult life. It may be associated with cysts in the liver and pancreas and berry aneurysms of the circle of Willis which cause subarachnoid haemorrhage. Many patients have no symptoms at all. Often the diagnosis is made by accident when an abdominal lump is found on routine palpation or ultrasound scanning.

Complications include the following:
1 Hypertension. This can be treated medically for many years.
2 Uraemia. At first this can be managed with restriction of protein. Later the patient may need dialysis, and ultimately may require a transplant.
3 Infection. It is rare for these cysts to become infected, but occasionally they do, and call for drainage. There is no other indication to drain these cysts: the so-called Rovsing operation has been shown to do more harm than good.

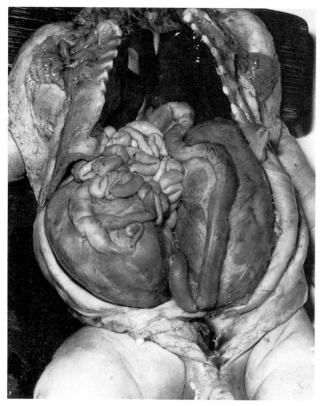

Fig. 4.26 Childhood polycystic disease. Courtesy of Mr J.H. Johnston.

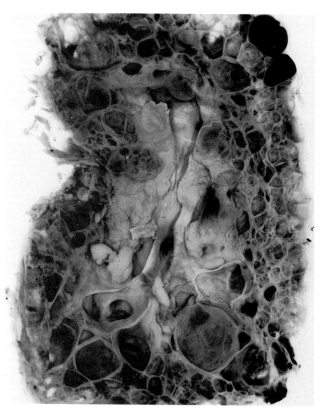

Fig. 4.27 Adult polycystic disease.

CONGENITAL DISORDERS OF THE RENAL TUBULES

Proximal tubules

A number of congenital errors involve the enzymes which transport amino acids across the mucosa of the bowel and the epithelium of the proximal renal tubule. The most important are as follows.

CYSTINURIA

Four amino acids are affected: cystine, ornithine, arginine and lysine ('coal'). The deficiency is inherited as a Mendelian autosomal recessive: only 3% of patients are

Cysteine

```
        COOH
         |
   H — C — NH₂
         |
   H — C — H
         |
        SH
- - - - - - - - - - - - -
        SH
         |
  H₃C — C — CH₃
         |
   H — C — NH₂
         |
        COOH
```

Penicillamine

Cystine

```
        COOH
         |
   H — C — NH₂
         |
   H — C — H
         |
         S
         |
         S
         |
   H — C — H
         |
   H — C — NH₂
         |
        COOH
```

Cysteine-Penicillamine

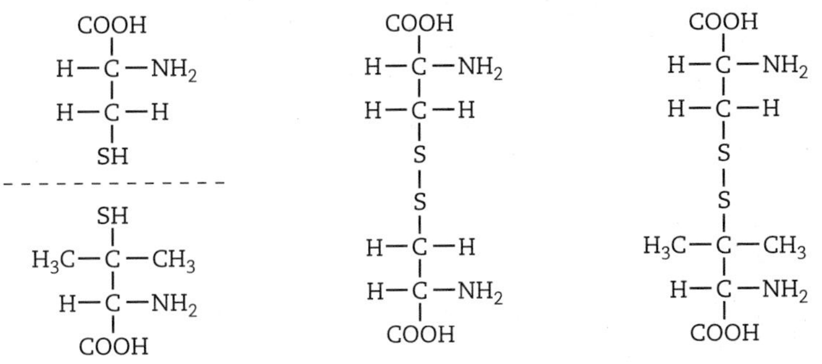

```
        COOH
         |
   H — C — NH₂
         |
   H — C — H
         |
         S
         |
         S
         |
  H₃C — C — CH₃
         |
   H — C — NH₂
         |
        COOH
```

Fig. 4.28 Cystine, cysteine and penicillamine.

homozygous. Cystine is poorly soluble in urine. Heterozygous patients lose about 500 mg/24 h in their urine: homozygous patients lose about 1 g/24 h and are bound to have urine supersaturated for cystine. Cystine stones are radiodense because of their sulphur content. Penicillamine binds the cystine in a soluble form and if combined with a high fluid input may prevent stones from forming and even dissolve those that are present (Fig. 4.28).

TRYPTOPHANE

In Hartnup disease tryptophane cannot be absorbed from the bowel, leading to nicotinamide deficiency, pellagra and cerebellar ataxia. In Fanconi's syndrome there is malabsorption of several amino acids as well as phosphate, and the disorder is accompanied by proteinuria and acidosis.

RENAL GLYCOSURIA

Here the tubules fail to reabsorb glucose which appears in the urine even when the blood sugar is normal. It is quite harmless but has to be distinguished from diabetes mellitus.

PHOSPHATE

If the tubules fail to reabsorb phosphate from the glomerular filtrate the result is vitamin D resistant rickets.

Distal renal tubules

RENAL TUBULAR ACIDOSIS

Disease of the distal tubule may make it unable to pump out hydrogen ions and the kidney cannot form an acid urine and loses potassium, phosphate, sulphate and other organic acids. The resulting low plasma bicarbonate increases the proportion of calcium which is not bound to protein, so more calcium escapes in the filtrate where it is precipitated in the tubules, leading to speckled calcification — nephrocalcinosis. At first these patients have normal glomerular function, but the loss of calcium and phosphate leads to osteomalacia. The diagnosis is made by the acid load test (see p. 36) and the remedy is potassium bicarbonate or citrate and additional vitamin D.

Collecting tubules

A sex-linked Mendelian recessive gene in males prevents collecting tubules from responding to the pituitary antidiuretic hormone — nephrogenic diabetes insipidus. Continued diuresis may lead to dehydration, severe enough to cause brain damage in the baby and gross dilatation of the kidneys and ureters.

Acquired disorders of the renal tubules

Obstructive uropathy

Back-pressure atrophy of the renal papillae is often seen in chronic obstruction. Glomerular filtration may be more or less unaffected, but the kidney is no longer able to acidify or concentrate the urine. The urine from the obstructed side is pale and has a fixed specific gravity. When both kidneys have been obstructed for a long time the patient may become severely dehydrated (see p. 202).

Sickle cell disease

In the sickle cell trait, even though there may never be a crisis, small vessels in the renal papilla may become blocked by the malformed red cells. The result is a series of ischaemic changes which result in an inability of the tubules to concentrate or acidify the urine. Microscopic haematuria is commonly present.

FURTHER READING

Anderson GA, Degroot D, Lawson RK (1993) Polycystic renal disease. *Urology* **42**: 358.
Blandy JP, Fowler CG (1996) *Kidney and Ureter — congenital abnormalities. Urology*, 2nd edn. Oxford, Blackwell Science, pp. 85–106.
Forget BC (1988) Sickle cell anemia and associated hemoglobinopathies. In: Wyngaarden JB, Smith LH, Bennett JC (eds) *Cecil Textbook of Medicine*. 19th edn. Philadelphia, WB Saunders, pp. 888–893.
Osathanondh V, Potter EL (1964) Pathogenesis of polycystic kidneys. Type 1 due to hyperplasia of interstitial portions of collecting tubules. *Arch Pathol* **77**: 466.
Saggar-Malik AK, Jeffery S, Patton MA (1994) Autosomal dominant polycystic kidney disease. *Br Med J* **308**: 1183.
Stein R, Ikoma F, Salge S, Miyanga T, Mori Y (1996) Pyeloplasty in hydronephrosis: examination of surgical results from a morphological point of view. *Int J Urol* **3**: 348.

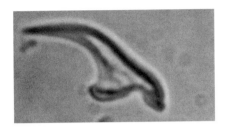

The Kidney: Trauma

PENETRATING INJURIES

The kidney may be injured by a bullet or knife wound and in such low velocity injuries the kidney can usually be repaired. In high velocity missile injuries the blast devitalizes a large sphere of tissue. If the kidney is within this sphere it must be removed or else there is likely to be fatal secondary haemorrhage.

CLOSED INJURIES

Closed injuries of the kidney are often seen in sport. To damage the kidney the blow has to be quite severe and often fractures the lower ribs and tips of the transverse processes of the lumbar vertebrae (Fig. 5.1).

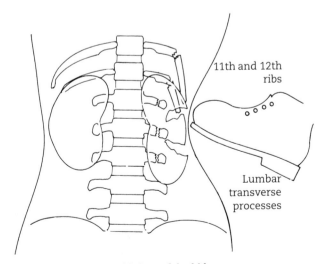

11th and 12th ribs

Lumbar transverse processes

Fig. 5.1 The mechanism of closed injury of the kidney.

There are three grades of closed renal injury (Fig. 5.2):

1   The parenchyma is split, causing haematuria and a surrounding haematoma, but the bleeding soon stops and the parenchyma heals completely within a few weeks.

2   The kidney splits into several fragments. Again, the thin strong bag of Gerota's fascia limits the expansion of the haematoma. The bleeding usually stops spontaneously and the kidney heals without any obvious sequel.

3   There is in addition a tear of the main renal artery or vein causing massive bleeding.

HISTORY

There is a story of an injury to the loin followed by haematuria.

SIGNS

On admission the patient is carefully examined to rule out pneumothorax, and internal bleeding into the chest or peritoneal cavity from associated injury to the liver or spleen. Every patient is admitted for observation because there is no way of telling how severe the original laceration of the kidney is, or how it is going to progress during the next few hours.

The chest is X-rayed. An emergency intravenous urogram (IVU) is performed not so much to show the type of the injury, but to make sure there is a kidney on the other side. The patient is then kept under close observation, the pulse, blood pressure and abdominal girth being recorded at regular intervals. Every specimen of urine is saved for inspection.

Nearly all these patients get steadily better. The colour of the blood in successive specimens of urine becomes less and less bright and the patient remains well.

But one cannot predict that this will happen all the time. Every so often things go wrong: there is a rising pulse, falling blood pressure and abdominal distension suggesting internal bleeding. The most useful investigation at this stage is a renal angiogram. This may identify the artery which is bleeding, and allow it to be plugged with gelfoam or chopped muscle injected through the catheter (Fig. 5.3). If this is not possible, or if the patient is obviously deteriorating, laparotomy must not be delayed.

The kidney is approached through a midline incision. The surgeon first secures the aorta and renal vessels before opening the perirenal fascia, which, until then, will have been limiting the bleeding by tamponade. Once the renal artery is secured and the clot evacuated, it may be possible to repair the damage but more often a nephrectomy is needed.

Recently it has become more common to ask for a computed tomography (CT) scan in the early investigation of such patients. This can be positively confusing. The appearance of the ruptured kidney in the CT scan can be frightening, but

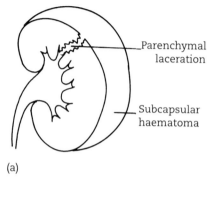
(a) Parenchymal laceration / Subcapsular haematoma

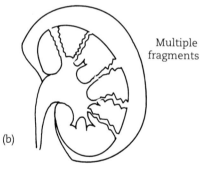
(b) Multiple fragments

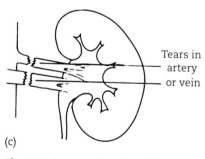
(c) Tears in artery or vein

Fig. 5.2 Three grades of renal injury.

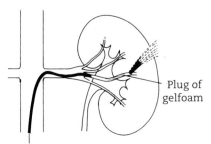

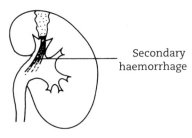

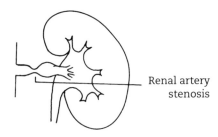

Plug of gelfoam

Angiographic catheter

Fig. 5.3 Bleeding from a segmental artery can be blocked by injection of gelfoam through an angiography catheter.

Secondary haemorrhage

Fig. 5.4 Secondary haemorrhage.

Renal artery stenosis

Fig. 5.5 Renal artery stenosis.

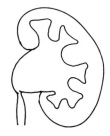

Fig. 5.7 Hydronephrosis.

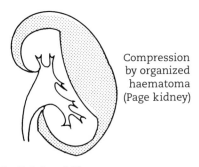

Compression by organized haematoma (Page kidney)

Fig. 5.6 Page kidney.

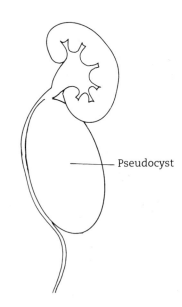

Pseudocyst

Fig. 5.8 Pseudocyst or urinoma.

is not an indication for open surgery, and if the CT scan is performed after the patient has started to deteriorate it may cause dangerous delay.

FOLLOW-UP

Five important complications must be borne in mind:

1 Secondary haemorrhage. When there has been a severe laceration the clot that is holding the pieces of kidney together may undergo lysis. Late secondary haemorrhage may occur at any time within the first 2 weeks, but is fortunately exceedingly rare when the initial tear in the kidney has only been a small one (Fig. 5.4).

2 Renal artery stenosis. A small laceration of the renal artery may heal with stenosis and cause hypertension (Fig. 5.5).

3   Page kidney. An organizing haematoma may form a thick tough shell around the kidney which then compresses it, makes it ischaemic and causes hypertension (Fig. 5.6).

4   Hydronephrosis. It is very rare to have documented evidence where a kidney was normal, and became hydronephrotic after injury. It is far more common for a hydronephrosis to be discovered after an injury. A distended balloon is more likely to burst than a floppy one and a distended hydronephrosis is more prone to trauma, but in the individual case the sequence of cause and effect is often open to question (Fig. 5.7).

5   Pseudocyst or urinoma. This is a very rare but potentially lethal complication. If the split in the renal pelvis allows urine to escape into the surrounding tissue it may form a large collection—a urinoma (Fig. 5.8) which becomes surrounded by a fibrous tissue wall which sometimes calcifies. The collection of urine inside the wall inevitably becomes infected and must not only be drained, but usually requires total excision.

FURTHER READING

Arnold EP (1972) Pararenal pseudocyst. *Br J Urol* **44**: 40.

Eastham JA, Wilson TG, Ahlering TE (1993) Urological evaluation and management of renal-proximity stab wounds. *J Urol* **150**: 1771.

McAndrew JD, Corriere JN (1994) Radiographic evaluation of renal trauma: evaluation of 1103 patients. *Br J Urol* **73**: 352.

Miller KS, McAninch JW (1995) Radiographic assessment of renal trauma: our 15-year experience. *J Urol* **154**: 352.

Page IH (1939) The production of persistent arterial hypertension by cellophane and perinephritis. *J Am Med Assoc* **113**: 2046.

Thall EH, Stone NN, Cheng DL *et al.* (1996) Conservative management of penetrating and blunt type III renal injuries. *Br J Urol* **77**: 512.

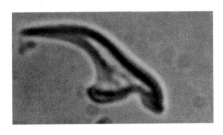

The Kidney: Inflammation

IMMUNOLOGICAL DISORDERS

Anything can act as an antigen either by itself or in combination with various peptides, and the list of antigens that can cause allergic inflammation in the kidney is very long, ranging from simple chemicals such as penicillamine and butazolidine, to microorganisms such as *Streptococcus* and *Plasmodium malariae*. Even the patient's own DNA can act as the allergen.

In a healthy patient the immune defences react to an unwanted antigen by smothering it with insoluble complex, which is then scavenged by the reticuloendothelial system before it can reach the kidney. If there is too little antibody to smother the antigen completely, smaller soluble complexes are formed, which may get trapped between the slit-pores in the glomerulus, or in the arteriole of the stalk of the glomerulus—the mesangium.

NEPHROTIC SYNDROME

Soluble complexes cause little damage. A renal biopsy seldom shows anything wrong on light microscopy and even the electron microscope shows only minimal damage to the basement membrane (Fig. 6.1). However, this is enough to allow the filter to leak albumen and cholesterol with the result that the plasma oncotic pressure falls and water leaks into the interstitial space, causing widespread oedema. The leaked cholesterol streaks the oedematous kidneys with lipid.

Clinically the picture is one of gross oedema: usually seen in children who fortunately recover spontaneously, sometimes with a little help from steroids.

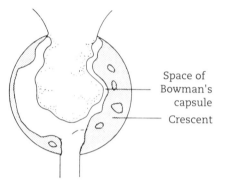

Fig. 6.1 Minimal change disease of the basement membrane.

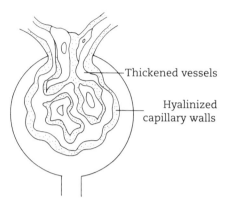

Fig. 6.2 Mesangiocapillary disease: inflammatory exudate in the mesangium and the glomerular tuft.

Fig. 6.3 Extracapillary proliferative disease: exudate fills up Bowman's capsule.

NEPHRITIC SYNDROME

The situation changes dramatically if the soluble complex fixes complement. This sets off the cascade of inflammation which results in the perforation of cell membranes, the release of histamine from mast cells and platelets, dilatation of blood vessels, and an influx of leucocytes. If the leucocytes stick in the mesangium or glomerular tuft the changes are usually reversible (Fig. 6.2) but if they burst out into the space of Bowman's capsule it becomes choked with cells and the outlook is far worse (Fig. 6.3).

The clinical picture of the nephritic syndrome is quite different from the nephrotic syndrome described above. There is a rapid onset with haematuria and hypertension and if the tubules are clogged with red and white cells there may be anuria. If the kidneys fail to clear themselves, they heal with scarring: the glomeruli are replaced by little hyaline spheres and the tubules are surrounded and compressed by scar tissue: the picture is described as end-stage renal disease which testifies to its grim outlook.

Five common clinical types of nephritic syndrome ought to be remembered.

1 Goodpasture syndrome. By a sad accident the basement membrane of the glomerulus has antigens similar to those of the pulmonary alveoli, and a lung infection can allow these to escape and get stuck in the filter where they fix complement. The nephritic syndrome is accompanied by haemoptysis.

2 Henoch–Schönlein nephritis. After a streptococcal infection a child has sudden pain in the abdomen and joints, with purpura and the nephritic syndrome.

3 Polyarteritis nodosa. Several different antigens can cause severe inflammation in the walls of arteries all over the body, including the kidney where the glomerular arterioles are affected by fibrinoid necrosis. Bowman's capsule is clogged with cells and the outlook is very bad.

4   Lupus nephritis. The antigen is the patient's own DNA whose soluble complexes are stuck in the glomeruli and fix complement.

5   Alport's syndrome. Here there is an inherited autosomal dominant condition which leads to the nephritic syndrome together with deafness, ocular abnormalities and polyneuropathy.

MATRIX DEPOSIT DISEASES

1   Diabetic nephropathy. An eosinophilic matrix is deposited in the glomerular arteriole causing its wall to thicken. There is loss of albumen and red cells, and hypertension follows.

2   Amyloidosis. Amyloid may be deposited in the glomerulus in both primary and secondary amyloidosis, giving a glassy eosinophilic deposit throughout the glomerulus and Bowman's capsule. The whole picture may be suddenly worsened by thrombosis of the renal vein.

3   Myelomatosis. In multiple myeloma the bone marrow produces an excess of immunoglobulins, and in 50% of patients light chain immunoglobulins appear in the urine as the Bence-Jones protein which coagulates when the urine is warmed to 50°C and dissolves again as it is warmed up even further.

ACUTE URINARY INFECTION

Ascending infection

Bacteria are always present in the distal urethra of either sex. If they reach the bladder and the ureteric valve is deficient reflux of urine will carry them up to the kidney where, if the renal papillae are of the compound type, infected urine will be injected into the parenchyma and cause inflammation (see p. 32).

Ascending infection is usually from an organism in the patient's own intestine, e.g. *Escherichia coli*, *Klebsiella*, *Streptococcus faecalis* or *Proteus mirabilis*. When a patient is given broad-spectrum antibiotics or sits around in hospital for any length of time, more dangerous and resistant organisms colonize the bowel. This is one of the main reasons why urologists are reluctant to use prophylactic antibiotics.

Haematogenous infection

Blood-borne infection may also carry microorganisms to the kidney to form multiple small abscesses. These are normally dealt with by the defence mechanisms and heal without significant scarring. They are often seen postmortem in patients who have had a terminal episode of bacteraemia. A previous scar in the kidney makes it more susceptible to such haematogenous infection. Important blood-borne infections include those due to staphylococci and *Mycobacterium tuberculo-sis* (see p. 66).

Factors predisposing to urinary infection (Fig. 6.4)

STAGNANT URINE

Urine is an excellent culture medium in which microorganisms multiply at body temperature unless the pool of urine is regularly and completely emptied out. Stagnant pools of urine occur under four circumstances.

1 Infrequent voiding. Some people empty their bladders very infrequently. As bacteria divide every 15 min, an inoculum of only 10 bacteria may in theory increase to 8×10^6 within 6 h. A practical way to prevent urinary infection is to persuade patients to empty their bladders every hour.

2 Mechanical obstruction. Obstruction occurs from a number of causes, e.g. hydronephrosis, a stone or an obstructing prostate gland. The end result is the same: there is a pool of stagnant urine which sooner or later becomes infected.

3 Undrained pockets of urine. Diverticula occur anywhere in the urinary tract, especially in the bladder and kidney, forming a pool of urine that never empties out completely.

4 Dilated and refluxing ureters. Many conditions cause the ureters to become dilated: there may be obstruction, e.g. by a stone or a tumour, or the ureterovesi-cal valve may be deficient. The end result is the same—a pool of urine that is never completely drained out, and invites infection.

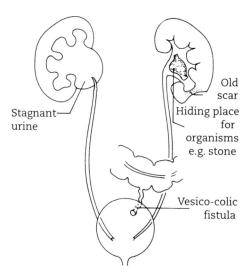

Fig. 6.4 Factors contributing to urinary infection.

HIDING PLACES FOR MICROORGANISMS

1 Stones. Stones are often crumbly, and a coating of slime between the crystals allows organisms to lurk, sheltered from antibiotics that cannot diffuse into the centre of the stone.

2 Very similar hiding places for bacteria are provided by dead tissue, e.g. in a cancer undergoing necrosis, or a foreign body such as a nylon stitch or a fragment of a catheter.

SOURCES OF REINFECTION

Microorganisms may be repeatedly injected into the urinary tract from a fistula into adjacent bowel, e.g. diverticular disease, cancer of the colon, and Crohn's disease of the small bowel (Fig. 6.5).

LOWERED RESISTANCE TO INFECTION

Impaired host resistance is seen in diabetes mellitus, acquired immune deficiency syndrome (AIDS), and therapeutic immunosuppression for transplantation or during cancer chemotherapy. It is a clinical commonplace to note that the symptoms of an ordinary urinary infection often begin a few days after an influenza-like illness which has impaired host resistance.

End result of urinary infection

Infection in the kidney, like infection anywhere else in the body can be followed by one of four processes (Fig. 6.6).

1 Resolution. This is the usual result. Most patients with bacterial infection in

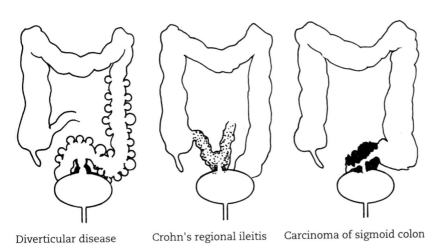

Diverticular disease   Crohn's regional ileitis   Carcinoma of sigmoid colon

Fig. 6.5 Infection from enterovesical fistulae.

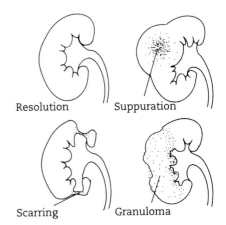

Resolution   Suppuration

Scarring   Granuloma

Fig. 6.6 Four possible outcomes from renal infection.

the bladder or kidney end up with an absolutely normal bladder and an undamaged kidney.

2 Suppuration. When the kidney is obstructed the entire kidney may be converted into a bag of pus — pyonephrosis. A minor form of this is seen when one calix is obstructed — pyocalix. Suppuration after haematogenous infection may cause an abscess in the renal cortex which spreads into the surrounding fat to cause a renal carbuncle (see p. 65).

3 Scarring. Scarring occurs when there has been both obstruction and infection: it may be diffuse — interstitial nephritis — or localized, to produce a deeply pitted scar in the parenchyma (see reflux nephropathy below).

4 Granuloma. Infection by organisms which cause chronic inflammation elsewhere, e.g. tuberculosis, brucellosis and actinomycosis, cause granuloma in the kidney. There are also a group of unusual granulomas which follow infection with *Escherichia coli* (see p. 69).

REFLUX NEPHROPATHY

Many children are born with defective valves at the entry of the ureters into the bladder, especially when there are other congenital anomalies such as duplex kidney or ureterocele (see p. 43). Urine is forced back up the ureter to the kidney. When, in addition, compound papillae do not have effective valves to protect the collecting tubules, urine is forced into the parenchyma. Uninfected urine probably causes little harm, but infected urine sets up acute inflammation which is followed by the typical deeply pitted scars of reflux nephropathy which become more pronounced as the rest of the kidney continues to grow. Compound papillae are usually found at the upper and lower poles of the kidney so it is here that the scarring of reflux nephropathy is most marked (Fig. 6.7).

The diagnosis is made by a micturating cystogram (see p. 20) or ultrasound scan using aerated water in the bladder which shows up on scanning. Three grades of reflux are recognized (Fig. 6.8). In grade I and II, where the reflux is not severe,

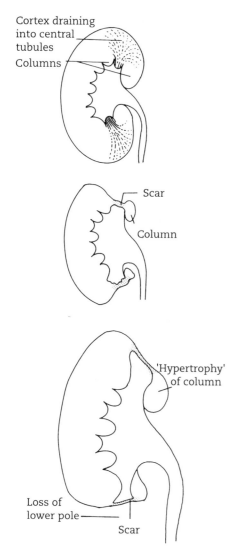

Fig. 6.7 Formation of the pitted scars of reflux nephropathy.

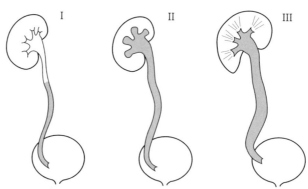

Fig. 6.8 Three grades of reflux.

the urine can usually be kept sterile with a small daily dose of an antimicrobial such as trimethoprim and it is safe to wait for the valve to mature and become competent.

In grade III, where the reflux is gross, it may be impossible to keep the urine sterile, or there is repeated breakthrough infection, and it may be better to perform an operation to prevent reflux. The most simple of these is to inject a small amount of collagen paste through a cystoscope under the mucosa of the ureteric orifice to change its opening into a crescent (Fig. 6.9). When the ureters are very dilated it may be necessary to reimplant the ureter through a long tunnel between the urothelium and muscle of the wall of the bladder (Fig. 6.10).

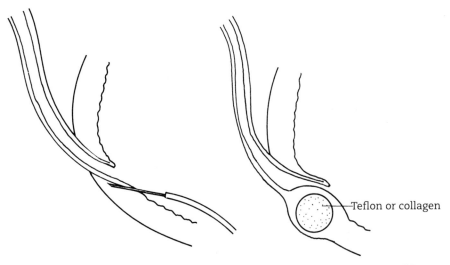

Teflon or collagen

Fig. 6.9 A blob of Teflon paste or collagen is injected under the urothelium of the ureteric orifice.

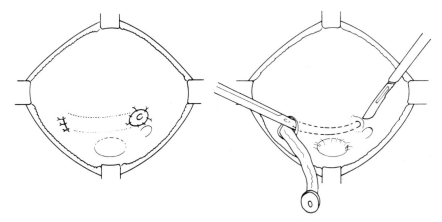

Fig. 6.10 Reimplantation of the ureter using Cohen's method.

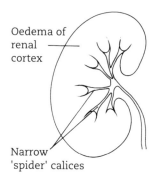

Oedema of renal cortex

Narrow 'spider' calices

Fig. 6.11 IVU in acute infection.

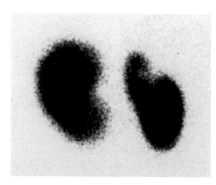

Fig. 6.12 DMSA renogram in acute infection showing lack of uptake of the isotope in a pyramid of the left kidney. Courtesy of Dr Neil Garvie.

COMPLICATIONS OF URINARY TRACT INFECTION

ACUTE RENAL FAILURE

Whether blood- or urine-borne the immediate effect on the parenchyma is like inflammation anywhere else: the kidney becomes hyperaemic and swollen, and may lose its function. The patient has pain in the loin and the kidney is tender on palpation. The intravenous urogram (IVU) may show no excretion of contrast, and the outline of the kidney and border of the psoas muscle are made fuzzy by oedema, which compresses the necks of the calices (Fig. 6.11). A dimercapto succinic acid (DMSA) renogram typically shows loss of uptake of the isotope in one or more pyramids. There may still be complete recovery (Fig. 6.12).

SEPTICAEMIA

The most serious of all the complications of acute urinary tract infection is septicaemia. There is only a very thin layer of tissue between the blood vessels of the kidney and the lumen of the urinary tract, and whenever there is an increase in pressure in the lumen microorganisms are easily forced directly into the veins and lymphatics of the kidney.

The organisms most likely to reach the bloodstream are Gram-negative bacilli, which contain lipid-A endotoxin. This releases kinins which make small blood vessels dilate and become leaky, depress the function of the cardiac muscle, and stimulate the hypothalamus to cause fever. Gram-negative septicaemia may occur after any urological operation without warning. There is at first a brief warning stage when the peripheral circulation is dilated, the patient has rigors, fever and a bounding pulse. The face and limbs are flushed and warm. Within half an hour this picture alters dramatically. The blood pressure falls to an almost unrecordable level. There is vasoconstriction of peripheral vessels and the limbs are cold: the patient looks as though he has suffered a myocardial infarct (Fig. 6.13).

Management

You have no time to lose. Summon help from the team in the Intensive Therapy Unit. Confirm the diagnosis by getting a needle into a vein while you still can find one (which may not be easy). Send blood for culture. Through the same needle inject a massive dose of the most appropriate antibiotic.

The choice of antibiotic may be obvious from the preoperative cultures of the urine, but if there is no bacteriological information, ask your colleagues in the hospital microbiology department to advise you as to the most likely cause of septicaemia and the most appropriate antibiotic.

Set up a saline infusion. Insert a central venous catheter to monitor the pressure in the right heart and then give enough plasma-expander to return the

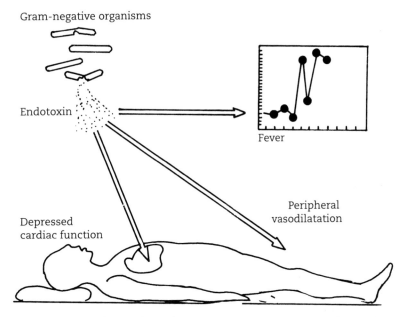

Fig. 6.13 Gram-negative septicaemia.

central venous pressure to normal. This may need 5 or 10 litres of fluid, and unless the central pressure is carefully monitored you may overload the heart.

Improvement usually takes place within 1 h, and within 2 h the peripheral vessels have recovered their tone and the lost fluid begins to return to the circulation. There is now a theoretical risk of overloading the circulation and precipitating heart failure. Usually natural diuresis quickly gets rid of the surplus fluid, but a diuretic or even venesection is sometimes needed.

When the patient has been resuscitated the underlying urological problem can be considered. Any localized pocket of infected urine must be drained, e.g. by percutaneous nephrostomy, emptying the bladder or draining an abscess.

STONE

Stones can form within weeks of an episode of infection. They may form upon a sloughed papilla (see p. 66) or bacterial debris in the urinary tract (Fig. 6.14). Infection with a urea-splitting organism such as *Proteus mirabilis* promotes the formation of a stone (see p. 75).

SUPPURATION

Blood-borne infection of the renal parenchyma begins as a collection of little abscesses which coalesce into an inflammatory mass which then liquefies into a collection of pus. In the days before antibiotics staphylococci from a boil in the

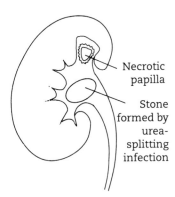

Necrotic papilla

Stone formed by urea-splitting infection

Fig. 6.14 Stones may form on a sloughed papilla or bacterial debris.

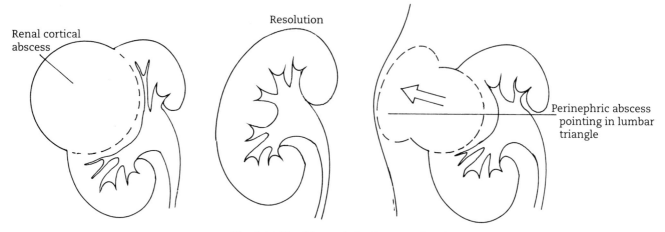

Fig. 6.15 Blood-borne infection may give rise to cortical infection which may resolve or proceed to an abscess.

skin were the usual organisms (Fig. 6.15). Today it is usually *Escherichia coli* from the urinary tract in people who are ill for some other reason, e.g. diabetes mellitus, or whose immune system has been suppressed by medication or AIDS.

Clinically the patient has a high fever and a swollen, tender kidney. When the infection is confined to the parenchyma there may be no pus cells or organisms in the urine. The X-rays show a soft tissue mass, and in the ultrasound and computed tomography (CT) scans the appearances may be confused with carcinoma. Clinical suspicion will suggest the right diagnosis, and it is confirmed by aspirating pus from the abscess. With effective antibiotic treatment these parenchymal abscesses usually resolve, with a surprising absence of scarring.

If diagnosed late, the abscess may burst into the perinephric fat, pointing in the loin through the lumbar triangle of Petit, where it is easily drained.

GRANULOMAS

Tuberculosis

For a time tuberculosis became so rare that we tended to forget about it. Today it is coming back, usually caused by the human variety of *Mycobacterium tuberculosis*. The primary focus in the lung sends blood-borne organisms to the kidney where they produce small tubercles which grow and erode into a papilla (Fig. 6.16). Patients may notice frequency of micturition and haematuria. The IVU may show an irregularity in a renal papilla which can be easy to overlook.

Later the abscess in the papilla enlarges, grows out to involve the rest of the pyramid, and may calcify (Fig. 6.17). The inflammation may narrow the neck of one or more calices which then fill with calcified debris (Fig. 6.18) and eventually the

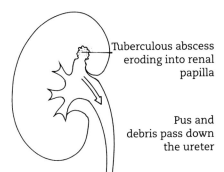

Tuberculous abscess eroding into renal papilla

Pus and debris pass down the ureter

Fig. 6.16 Tuberculous abscess in a renal papilla.

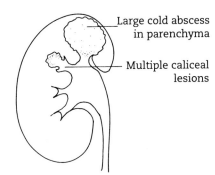

Large cold abscess in parenchyma

Multiple caliceal lesions

Fig. 6.17 Extension of the tuberculous abscess to the calix.

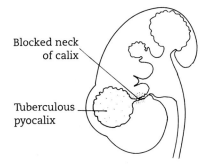

Blocked neck of calix

Tuberculous pyocalix

Fig. 6.18 Multiple tuberculous pyocalices.

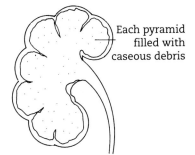

Each pyramid filled with caseous debris

Fig. 6.19 The cement kidney.

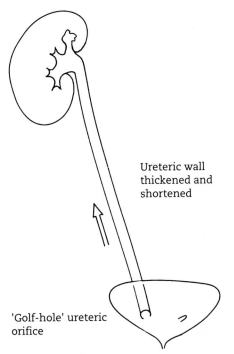

Ureteric wall thickened and shortened

'Golf-hole' ureteric orifice

Fig. 6.20 Shortening of the tuberculous ureter.

entire kidney can be converted into a bag of calcified caseation tissue which has a striking appearance in the plain X-ray—cement kidney (Fig. 6.19).

From the kidney the infection spreads down the ureter to the bladder. The ureter becomes stiff, oedematous and shortened so that the ureteric orifice is pulled up to give the appearance of a golf-hole (Fig. 6.20). Later on, as antituberculous chemotherapy begins to work and the granulomas in the wall of the ureter heal up, the ureter may become narrowed by scarring to cause hydronephrosis (Fig. 6.21).

In the bladder the early phase of tuberculosis may cause oedema, ulceration or polypi resembling a tumour on cystoscopy. Biopsy shows the characteristic tubercles, giant cells and acid-fast bacilli. The lesions in the bladder rapidly heal with treatment, but as with the ureter, scarring may cause the bladder to shrink with the result that the patient may have severe frequency of micturition.

Diagnosis

It needs suspicion to diagnose genitourinary tuberculosis. One good rule is to insist that every patient with pus in the urine, not explained by bacterial infection, must have tuberculosis excluded. Classically three early morning samples of urine are stained with auramine and examined under ultraviolet light, and in addition cultured on special Loewenstein–Jensen medium for up to 6 weeks. Guinea-pig inoculation is no longer used.

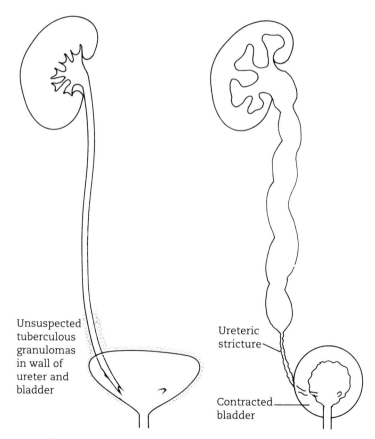

Unsuspected tuberculous granulomas in wall of ureter and bladder

Ureteric stricture

Contracted bladder

Fig. 6.21 Healing leading to obstruction of the ureter.

Treatment

Tuberculosis is a systemic disease. The patient often has active disease in the chest. The disease must be notified so that contacts can be traced. In practice this means you should summon the help of a colleague, usually a chest physician, who can treat the whole patient and will be expert in the dosage and details of combination chemotherapy. Treatment is usually started with rifampicin 450 mg, isonicotinic acid hydrazide (INAH) 300 mg, and ethambutol 800 mg daily for the first 3 months, followed by rifampicin and INAH for another 3–6 months. Today more cases are being found where the mycobacteria are resistant to these first-line antibiotics: another reason for getting expert help.

This does not mean that the urologist has handed over his or her responsibilities: each case must be carefully followed up. With very small lesions in one or two renal papillae one expects a complete resolution with, at worst, a fleck of calcification to mark the site of the tuberculous granuloma. Silent granulomas in the wall of the ureter may cause stenosis, and to detect this the intravenous pyelogram (IVP) or ultrasound must be repeated within 2 weeks of starting treatment. Early stenosis of the ureter may be prevented by means of a double-J splint for a few weeks, and so long as the sensitivity of the mycobacteria is known, steroids may assist in the prevention of scarring.

If a stricture does form up near the renal pelvis a pyeloplasty may be performed (see p. 128). When the narrowing is near the bladder the ureter may need to be reimplanted (see p. 133). If the entire length of the ureter is stenosed it can be replaced with ileum (see p. 172). A contracted bladder can be enlarged by one or other types of cystoplasty (see p. 173).

Unfortunately patients often come up at a stage when the kidney is too badly affected to recover useful function: in these cases, after preliminary treatment with antibiotics nephrectomy should be performed. Thanks to the efficacy of modern chemotherapy there is no longer any need to remove the ureter as well.

In males urinary tuberculosis may be accompanied by tuberculosis of the prostate, seminal vesicles, epididymes and vasa deferentia, while in women there may be involvement of the fallopian tubes and uterus.

Xanthogranuloma

This occurs around a renal calculus usually in association with *Proteus mirabilis* infection. There is a very strange granuloma, in which the histiocytes are stuffed with lipid, and the tissue resembles renal cell cancer in its bright yellow colour. The inflammation burrows into the tissues around the kidney (Fig. 6.22) as well as adjacent viscera, e.g. liver, colon and duodenum. The patient is always very ill, with fever and loss of weight. Antibiotics do not work: the mass must be removed.

Malacoplakia

This is another curious granuloma seen in the urinary tract which gives rise to

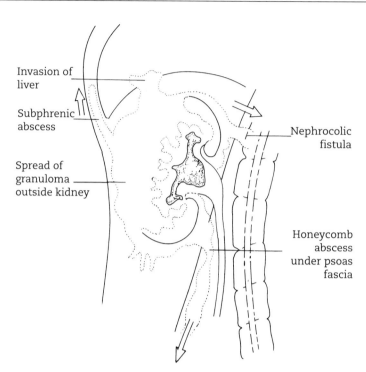

Fig. 6.22 Xanthogranuloma burrows into the surrounding tissues.

multiple abscesses and dense fibrosis. In the bladder and ureter it produces soft brown plaques which bleed easily, and may cause obstruction. It may respond to a prolonged course of trimethoprim.

Brucellosis

Brucella abortus or *B. melitensis* may cause a granuloma in the kidney that is very like tuberculosis, and behaves in a similar way. It occurs in communities where brucellosis is still rife in cattle. It can also involve the testis.

INTERSTITIAL NEPHRITIS, PYELONEPHRITIS, PAPILLARY NECROSIS

There is a spectrum of change in the kidney which may be caused by many things: at one end of the spectrum there is diffuse scarring throughout the renal parenchyma — interstitial nephritis. At the other end, the renal papilla undergoes necrosis and may become completely detached — papillary necrosis (Fig. 6.23).

INFECTION

Severe infection, particularly when combined with obstruction, can lead to

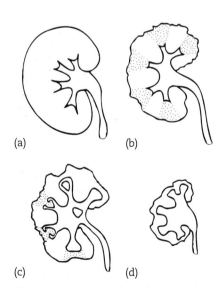

Fig. 6.23 Spectrum of changes in pyelonephritis.

interstitial nephritis, and in severe cases, to necrosis of the papilla especially when there is obstruction or some other underlying disorder such as diabetes mellitus.

ANALGESIC ABUSE

There have been a number of epidemics in which whole populations have taken to consuming large amounts of aspirin, phenacitin and similar analgesic medications: examples include the housewives of Newcastle (Australia), the watchmakers of Switzerland, and the motorcycle workers of Husqvarna in Sweden. There is every combination of interstitial nephritis and papillary necrosis.

BALKAN NEPHROPATHY

In isolated villages in the Balkans epidemics occur in which large numbers of people develop interstitial nephritis and papillary necrosis.

CHINESE HERBAL SLIMMING MEDICINES

Belgian ladies attending a fashionable slimming clinic were given an extract of *Aristolochia fang-ji* by mistake. They developed renal failure, and some went on to develop multifocal cancer (see p. 72). It has been suggested that perhaps a similar herb, *Aristolochia clematis*, may be responsible for Balkan nephropathy (see above).

GOUT AND NEPHROCALCINOSIS

The sharp needles of uric acid found in gout, and the crystals of calcium salts found

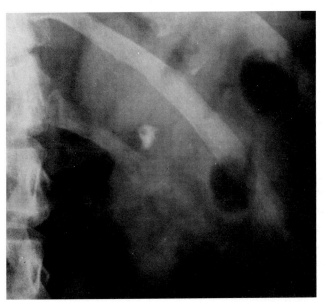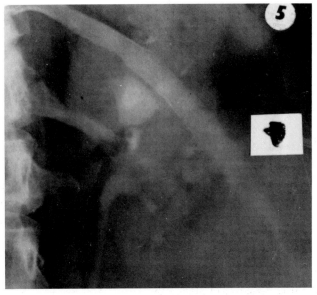

Fig. 6.24 Calcification on a dead papilla forming a stone which is blocking a calix.

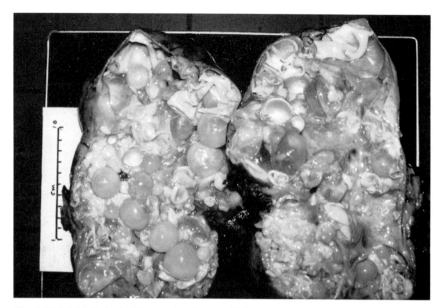

Fig. 6.25 Multiple hydatid cysts in a human kidney. Courtesy of Mr G. Ravi.

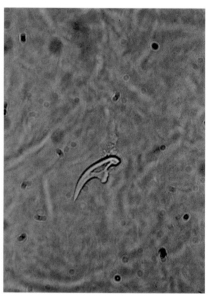

Fig. 6.26 Hooklet in fluid aspirated from a hydatid cyst. Courtesy of Professor J.D. Williams.

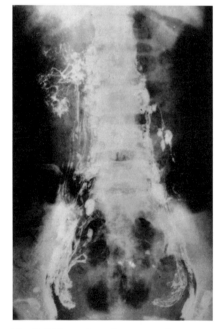

Fig. 6.27 Lymphangiogram and retrograde urogram showing connection with lymphatics of the kidney, in a case of chyluria. Courtesy of Mr Henry Yu.

in nephrocalcinosis are deposited in and around the renal tubules and may provoke scarring similar to interstitial nephritis.

CLINICAL FEATURES

Whatever the cause, the clinical features of interstitial nephritis are similar. There is loss of protein, progressive renal failure at first of the tubules, and later of the glomeruli. In most severe cases the sloughed renal papilla may become detached and pass down the ureter (causing obstruction) or remain and calcify in the kidney, to form a stone with a typically radiolucent centre (Fig. 6.24). Many of these patients come to dialysis, and several years later, the survivors are prone to develop multifocal transitional cell cancer involving the renal pelvis and calices (see p. 99).

HYDATID DISEASE

The tapeworm *Echinococcus granulosus* normally lives in sheep. Dogs eat uncooked sheep offal containing the worms, which thrive inside the dog, and shed eggs which collect on the dog's fur. Children fondle the dogs, forget to wash their hands, and swallow the ova. The eggs hatch out, and the worms burrow through the wall of the child's gut to reach the liver and kidney where they grow, multiply and form large collections of cysts. The cysts are multilocular. Their walls are more or less calcified, and the appearances are easily mistaken for cancer on ultrasound or CT scanning (Fig. 6.25). An immunoassay for a specific circulating antigen confirms the diagnosis. If, by mistake, the fluid inside the hydatid cyst is aspirated it will be found to be full of little hooklets (Fig. 6.26) but aspiration is avoided because it may spread the disease as well as precipitate an acute allergic attack.

After a course of albendazole the affected kidney should be removed, taking great care not to spill the cysts. The kidney is approached through the loin and the wound protected with packs soaked in 1% formalin or hypertonic saline. The biggest cysts are then aspirated, and the fluid replaced with 1% formalin or hypertonic saline, reaspirated, and then only when there is no risk of the kidney bursting, is it removed *en bloc*. If the tiny tapeworms inside the cysts are spilt they give rise to local recurrence which may be inoperable.

CHYLURIA

In the Far East fistulae form between the perirenal lymphatics and the renal pelvis, and lymphangiography shows a communication between them (Fig. 6.27). Sometimes it is possible to prove that the cause is infestation with the roundworm *Wuchereria bancroftii* which is transmitted by mosquitoes. Fat absorbed from food is continually lost into the urine which from its content of fat and blood, comes to resemble anchovy sauce. Although the continuous loss of protein may lead to starvation, this is rare, and usually the condition does not need any treatment at all.

Silver nitrate can be injected through a ureteric catheter to seal off the communications. If this fails, the kidney may be dissected from the lymphatics, which must all be carefully ligated.

FURTHER READING

Aaronson IA (1995) Current status of the 'sting'—an American perspective. *Br J Urol* **75**: 121.

Asscher AW (1987) Interstitial nephritis and urinary tract infection. In: Weatherall DJ, Ledingham JGG, Warrell DA (eds) *Oxford Textbook of Medicine*, 2nd edn, vol. 2. Oxford, Oxford University Press, pp. 18.67–80.

Childs S (1992) Current diagnosis and treatment of urinary infections. *Urology* **40**: 295.

Edwards JD (1993) Management of septic shock. *Br Med J* **306**: 1661.

Lebowitz RL (1992) The detection and characterization of vesicoureteric reflux in the child. *J Urol* **148**: 1640.

Marsh FP (1987) Toxic nephropathies. In: Weatherall DJ, Ledingham JGG, Warrell DA (eds) *Oxford Textbook of Medicine*, 2nd edn, vol. 2. Oxford, Oxford University Press, pp. 18.108–118.

Mason PD, Pusey CD (1994) Glomerulonephritis: diagnosis and treatment. *Br Med J* **309**: 1157.

Rushton HG, Majid M (1992) Dimercaptosuccinic acid renal scintigraphy for the evaluation of pyelonephritis and scarring: a review of experimental and clinical studies. *J Urol* **148**: 1726.

Smellie JM, Poulton A, Prescod NP (1994) Retrospective study of children with renal scarring associated with reflux and urinary infection. *Br Med J* **308**: 1193.

Watkins PJ (1982) ABC of diabetes: nephropathy. *Br Med J* **285**: 627.

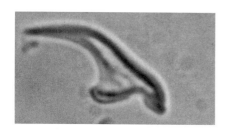

Urinary Calculi

Operations for the stone were well known in the time of Hippocrates, whose Oath enjoined young doctors to leave 'cutting for the stone' to those who were properly trained to do it. The incidence of stone varies in different populations. In the West there has been a steady rise in the incidence of calculi in the kidney and ureter, interrupted only by two World Wars, from which it is argued that stones reflect affluence and overfeeding with refined sugar and protein. Stones are more common in those whose work causes them to become dehydrated and form more concentrated urine. It is probable that the incidence of bladder stones in children in underdeveloped countries is an echo of infantile diarrhoeal diseases and dehydration.

A stone consists of crystalline material arranged on an organic scaffold like ferro-concrete or fibreglass (Fig. 7.1). We know little about the organic scaffold, but a lot about the formation of the crystals.

Salt added to water continues to dissolve until no more will do so: this is the saturation concentration, which is measured by the solubility product of the concentration of ions making up the salt (Fig. 7.2). In urine a metastable solution forms which does not precipitate crystals, even though the saturation concentration has been exceeded, unless the solution is left undisturbed for a long time, or is seeded with a nucleus on which stones can precipitate. If the concentration exceeds that of the metastable region, crystals precipitate to make their own nuclei—nucleation. Human urine is always metastable with respect to the main crystalline components of stones, calcium and oxalate.

The metastable state is influenced by temperature, the presence of colloids, the rate of flow of the urine, the concentration of the solutes and the presence of anything which can act as a nucleus, e.g. dead papillae (see p. 71), necrotic carcinoma, a non-absorbable suture, a fragment of catheter, or a previously existing fragment of stone (Fig. 7.3).

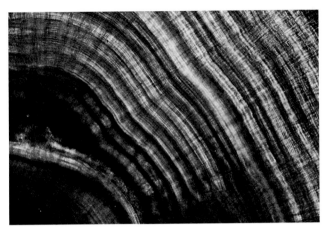

Fig. 7.1 Cross-section of a stone showing its laminations.

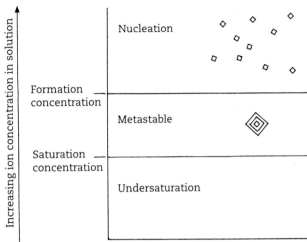

Fig. 7.2 Increasing ion concentration in a fluid such as urine.

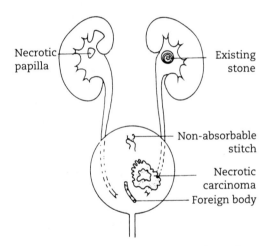

Fig. 7.3 Many conditions can act as a nucleus for stone formation.

The pH of the urine may be important in the formation of calculi: magnesium ammonium phosphate is insoluble in alkaline urine, and is precipitated by infection with *Proteus mirabilis* and other urea-splitting organisms. Uric acid is insoluble in an acid urine, but may dissolve if the urine is made alkaline.

All crystals prefer to be undisturbed if they are to grow, so calculi tend to form wherever there is stagnant urine, as in a ureterocele, a diverticulum, a hydronephrosis or a chronically obstructed bladder.

SUPERSATURATION STONES

The best examples of supersaturation stones are cystine and uric acid.

CYSTINE

In cystinuria there is a congenital (Mendelian recessive) defect in the enzymes necessary for the transport of cystine, ornithine, arginine and lysine in the proximal tubule (see p. 50). Homozygotes pass about 1 g/24h, heterozygotes about 0.5 g. Cystine is more soluble in an alkaline urine: penicillamine produces a soluble penicillamine–cysteine molecule (see p. 51).

URIC ACID

Uric acid is a weak acid, and is only half-ionized in urine of pH 5.75. Increasing the pH means that a much greater proportion is in the soluble ionized form: if the urine is allowed to become acid, most of it will be precipitated. An excess of uric acid occurs when there is a primary defect of metabolism of uric acid (as in gout) or rapid catabolism of protein, e.g. after cancer chemotherapy. Uric acid stones occur whenever the urine is very concentrated and very acid, as is seen in dehydration and in patients with ulcerative colitis and ileostomies. In addition the distal tubule in some patients is not able to form an alkaline urine, and they tend to have uric acid stones.

Treatment consists of providing a large water input, together with bicarbonate to keep the urine alkaline, and perhaps allopurinol to inhibit xanthine oxidase and prevent the formation of uric acid.

CALCIUM STONES

Most non-infective stones are made of calcium oxalate and/or calcium phosphate.

Oxalate

PRIMARY (HEPATIC) OXALURIA

An excess of oxalate is formed in primary hyperoxaluria, because of an inherited liver enzyme deficiency (either of glyoxalate carboligase, or δ-glycerate dehydrogenase) leading to an excess of oxalate in the urine which precipitates in the collecting tubules and eventually leads to renal failure (Fig. 7.4). Unfortunately a transplanted kidney suffers the same fate, but a combined liver and kidney transplant can be successful.

SECONDARY (ILEAL) OXALURIA

Hyperoxaluria also occurs in diseases of the terminal ileum where bile acids are

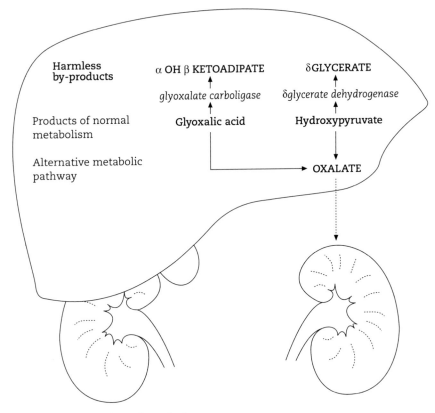

Fig. 7.4 Primary or hepatic oxaluria.

normally absorbed. If bile acids are not reabsorbed and recycled in the liver to be added to bile, then dietary fat cannot be emulsified, and remains in the bowel where it forms an insoluble soap with dietary calcium (Fig. 7.5). This in turn leaves an excess of dietary oxalate which is absorbed, excreted in the urine, and forms a stone. This type of hyperoxaluria may be prevented by giving cholestyramine (which binds the oxalate in the gut) and by avoiding food rich in oxalate such as tea, chocolate, coffee, spinach and rhubarb.

Hypercalciuria

An excess of calcium in the urine (i.e. >350 mg/24 h in males, >300 mg/24 h in females) may be a cause of stones in some males. There are three types:

1 Renal, where there is decreased renal tubular reabsorption of calcium. Little can be done about this.

2 Absorptive, where too much calcium is absorbed from the bowel. Many types of treatment were formerly given to diminish this, e.g. cellulose phosphate was

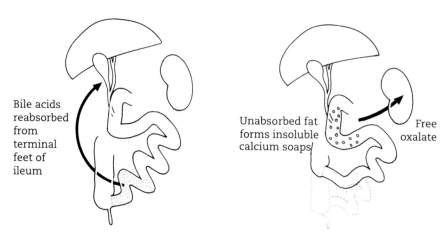

Fig. 7.5 Ileal oxaluria.

given to precipitate calcium salts in the bowel: patients were advised to give up milk products as well as all those rich in oxalate (see p. 77). In addition magnesium salts were given to try to keep calcium particles in suspension in the urine. In fact, all these treatments were ineffective and it is far more important to keep the urine dilute by drinking plenty of water, and perhaps encourage this with a small dose of a diuretic such as frusemide.

3 Resorptive hypercalciuria, where an excess of calcium is absorbed from the bones, depends on the function of the parathyroid glands.

Most of the calcium in the blood is bound to protein, only a small fraction is in solution, and of this an even smaller part is ionized. The product of the ions [Ca $\times$ PO_4] is kept constant. If [Ca] is increased, then [PO_4] must fall, and vice versa. Parathyroid hormone encourages osteoclasts to dissolve bone and release calcium into the blood: the output of the hormone is regulated by the concentration of ionized [Ca]. There are three types of hyperparathyroidism as follows.

PRIMARY HYPERPARATHYROIDISM

For no known reason, the parathyroid glands start to secrete more parathyroid hormone than is needed with the result that calcium is reabsorbed from the skeleton and added to the blood. The plasma [Ca] rises and the plasma [PO_4] has to fall. The excess calcium enters the urine where it precipitates in the renal tubules as one form of nephrocalcinosis, or forms a stone in the renal tract (Fig. 7.6).

The diagnosis of primary hyperparathyroidism is usually made by the chance finding of an elevated [Ca] in the course of a routine blood test or in the investigation of a patient with a stone. It is very rare to find the classical changes of osteitis fibrosa cystica where massive collections of osteoclasts cause cystic cavities in bones and sometimes a pathological fracture. The finding of an elevated plasma

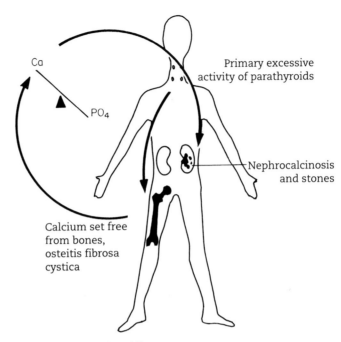

Fig. 7.6 Primary hyperparathyroidism.

[Ca] must always be double checked, and if confirmed, then the plasma parathyroid hormone is measured by radioimmunoassay.

SECONDARY HYPERPARATHYROIDISM

In chronic renal failure, phosphate is one of the metabolic products that are not adequately excreted, so the plasma [PO$_4$] rises, and the [Ca] has to fall. The [Ca] is precipitated in soft tissues as heterotopic calcification where it may cause joint stiffness and deafness. The parathyroids respond to the lowered [Ca] by secreting more parathyroid hormone, and all four glands become hyperplastic. Secondary hyperparathyroidism is still seen in patients undergoing dialysis for renal failure, but can largely be prevented by large doses of vitamin D which encourage the absorption of calcium from the bowel (Fig. 7.7).

TERTIARY HYPERPARATHYROIDISM

Here the overactive parathyroid glands seem not to know when to stop and in spite of extra vitamin D, keep on putting out far more parathyroid hormone than is needed to maintain a constant [Ca]. When this occurs they must be removed.

PARATHYROIDECTOMY

The four parathyroid glands are each about the size of a pea and lie behind and buried in the lateral lobes of the thyroid gland near the superior and inferior

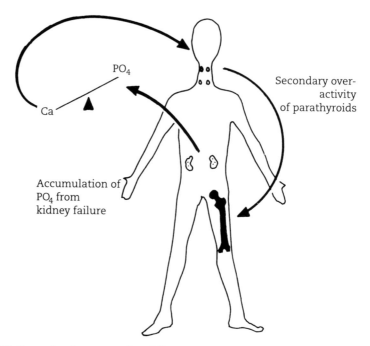

Fig. 7.7 Secondary hyperparathyroidism.

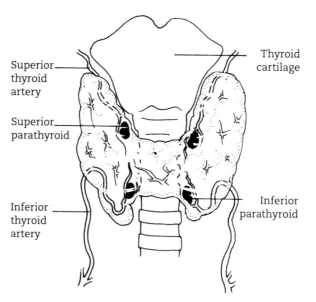

Fig. 7.8 Anatomical relations of the parathyroid glands.

thyroid arteries (Fig. 7.8). Primary hyperparathyroidism may be caused by an adenoma in one gland or hyperplasia of all four. The glands are localized by subtraction radioisotope scans, and at operation all four glands are confirmed by biopsy and frozen section. Occasionally a 'missing' parathyroid gland is found in the mediastinum.

FORMATION OF RENAL CALCULI

Tiny spheres of calcium phosphate are often found in normal collecting ducts — Carr's concretions. Collections of these gather near the tip of a papilla to form shining plaques easily seen with a nephroscope — Randall's plaques. When these become detached they may act as a nucleus for further stone formation (Fig. 7.9). A similar nucleus is formed by a necrotic renal papilla (see p. 71). From then on the stone continues to grow as layer after layer of calcium salts, together with a protein matrix, is laid down.

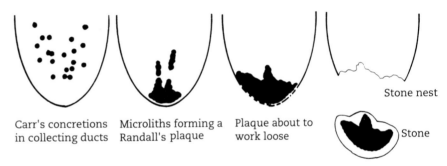

Carr's concretions in collecting ducts   Microliths forming a Randall's plaque   Plaque about to work loose   Stone nest   Stone

Fig. 7.9 Formation of calculus in a renal papilla.

Investigation of a calculus

Where is the stone, and is it likely to do any harm?
An intravenous urogram (IVU) will usually show where the stone is situated, and whether it is likely to get stuck and cause obstruction. The exceptions are those made of uric acid and cystine. Stones made of uric acid are completely radiolucent, and do not show in a plain radiograph, but they do cast an acoustic shadow on ultrasound scan and show up in a computed tomography (CT) scan. Stones made of cystine are faintly radio-opaque because of their sulphur content, and are always easily located with ultrasound or CT scan.

What is the cause of the stone, and can it be prevented?
Hyperparathyroidism must be ruled out by measuring the plasma [Ca]. The urine should be checked for infection especially with urea-splitting organisms. The

whole state of the urinary tract needs to be examined for possible collections of stagnant urine, and one must always consider the possibility that the stone may have formed on a non-absorbable suture or other foreign body.

MANAGEMENT OF A RENAL STONE

As a general rule the normal ureter will allow a stone to pass if it is less than 5 mm in diameter. Stones larger than this are likely to get stuck and should usually be removed.

When a stone is stuck it causes obstruction, but this rarely remains complete for very long, and soon the urine finds it way past the stone. If the urine also happens to be infected there is a risk that back-pressure will cause septicaemia (see p. 64) and/or obstructive nephropathy (see p. 64) so there is then an urgent necessity to overcome the obstruction either by an emergency percutaneous nephrostomy (see p. 19) or by passing a double-J splint from below. The infection cannot usually be eradicated if a stone is present because it shields microorganisms from antibiotics. Urea-splitting organisms will precipitate layers of magnesium ammonium phosphate (apatite) on any existing stone.

Methods for removing stones

EXTRACORPOREAL SHOCK-WAVE LITHOTRIPSY

Shock waves travel through water. Different types of lithotriptors generate shock waves, and focus them on the stone by means of X-rays or ultrasonic scanners. The shock waves break the stone up into fragments small enough to pass down the ureter.

Many different types of lithotriptor are available, differing in the method by which the shock wave is generated and the stone is localized. To generate the shock wave some use a spark-plug, others an array of piezo-ceramic shock emittors (Fig. 7.10). Some localize the stone with ultrasound, others use X-rays.

However the stone is broken up, the little fragments have to go down the ureter. There they may cause temporary obstruction — the *steinstrasse* — and diclofenac may be needed for ureteric colic (Fig. 7.11). But with a large fluid throughput the steinstrasse usually clears within a few days.

It may be necessary to repeat the lithotripsy several times, according to the density of the stones. For larger stones extracorporeal shock-wave lithotripsy (ESWL) is often combined with percutaneous nephrolithotomy (PCNL).

PERCUTANEOUS NEPHROLITHOTOMY

After placing a needle under X-ray or ultrasound control into the renal pelvis, a

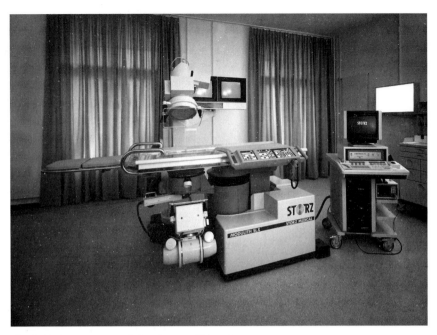

Fig. 7.10 Extracorporeal shock-wave lithotripsy.

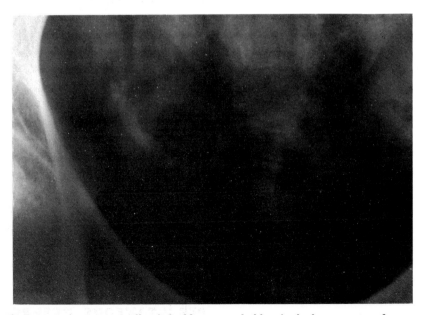

Fig. 7.11 Steinstrasse—collection of fragments held up in the lower ureter after ESWL.

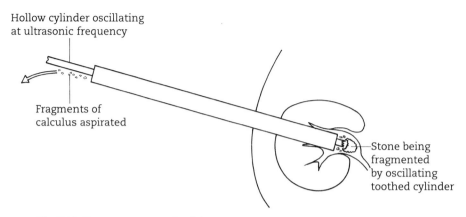

Hollow cylinder oscillating
at ultrasonic frequency

Fragments of
calculus aspirated

Stone being
fragmented
by oscillating
toothed cylinder

Fig. 7.12 Percutaneous nephrolithotomy.

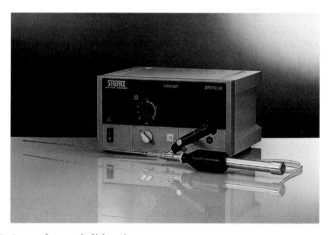

Fig. 7.13 Storz ultrasonic lithotriptor.

guide-wire is passed, and the needle withdrawn. A series of dilators of increasing size are then passed over the guide-wire until a track has been made into the kidney big enough to admit a working sheath, through which instruments can be passed (Fig. 7.12). The stone is now examined with a nephroscope, and broken up with one of several ingenious gadgets: one emits a stream of sparks which cracks the stone; another does the same thing with a Q-switched laser; a third grinds the stone to powder with a toothed cylinder oscillated at ultrasonic frequency; and a fourth uses a miniature jack-hammer to break up the stone. A variety of forceps are then available to pick out the bits (Fig. 7.13).

DOUBLE-J URETERIC STENT

To help the ureter to dilate, and encourage the passage of the fragments of stone after ESWL, a double-J stent is often passed up the ureter over a guide-wire intro-

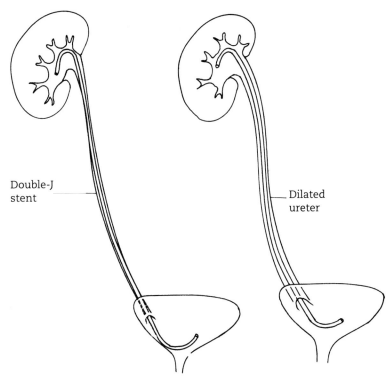

Double-J
stent

Dilated
ureter

Fig. 7.14 A double-J stent helps the ureter to dilate.

duced through a flexible or rigid cystoscope (Fig. 7.14). When this is done the double-J splint can be left in for several months, but there is a risk that the double-J splint may itself act as a nucleus for stone formation, and strict precautions have to be taken to follow the patient up and make sure the splint is retrieved within a reasonable time.

Ureteroscopy

A ureteroscope may be passed up the ureter to break up and remove small stones that are stuck in the ureter: miniature versions of the Q-switched laser and jack-hammer are available for this procedure (Fig. 7.15).

Stones in common sites

STONE IN A CALIX

Caliceal stones seldom cause any trouble and can as a rule be safely kept under

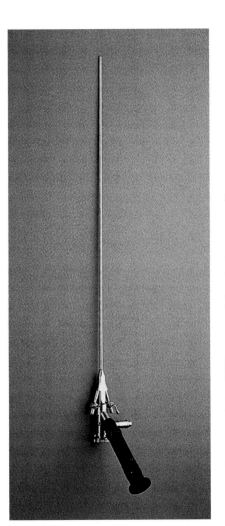

Fig. 7.15 Storz ureteroscope.

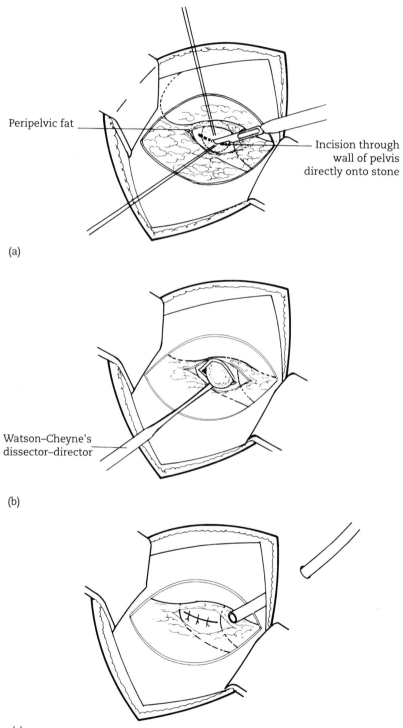

Peripelvic fat

Incision through
wall of pelvis
directly onto stone

(a)

Watson–Cheyne's
dissector–director

(b)

(c)

Fig. 7.16 Pyelolithotomy.

observation. Very occasionally they seem to cause pain and may be fragmented by ESWL.

STONE IN THE RENAL PELVIS

A stone in the renal pelvis which is more than 5 mm diameter will probably get stuck when it tries to go down the ureter and should be got rid of by ESWL or

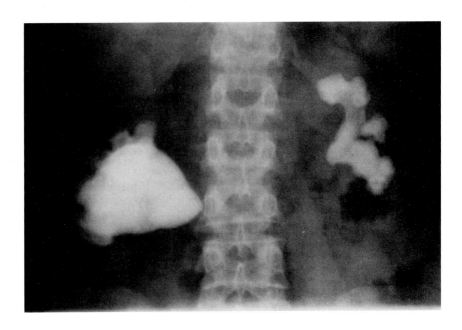

Fig. 7.17 Staghorn stones may fill the entire collecting system.

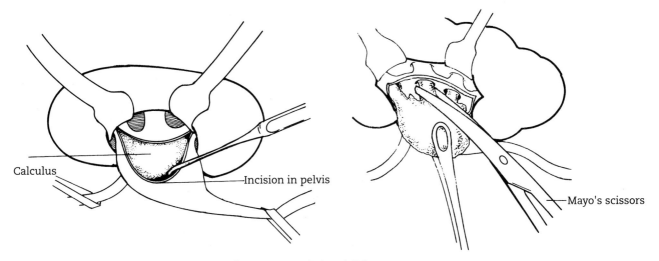

Fig. 7.18 Extended pyelolithotomy.

PCNL before the patient has any symptoms. These renal pelvic stones can cause repeated attacks of renal colic and haematuria, and may be associated with infection.

Stones in the pelvis used to be removed by pyelolithotomy. The kidney was approached through the 12th rib tip incision, and mobilized to give access to the renal pelvis, which was opened between stay stitches: the stone was removed, the pelvis closed and the wound closed with a drain (Fig. 7.16).

STAGHORN STONES

Stones sometimes fill the entire pelvis and nearly all the calices (Fig. 7.17), usually in the presence of *Proteus mirabilis* infection. The body of the stone is usually removed by PCNL while the outlying bits in the calices are broken up with extracorporeal lithotripsy in a series of sessions. This can require the patient to undergo a long series of operations, even though none of them are very major, and at the end of the day small bits of stone are often left behind. From time to time there is a case to be made to perform extended pyelolithotomy (Fig. 7.18).

Here the kidney is approached through the loin, fully mobilized, its renal artery taped (for safety) and the bloodless plane between the renal pelvis and parenchyma opened up to allow the parenchyma to be lifted up, after which the pelvis is laid open up from the upper to the lower calix. The stone is then extracted completely, and the kidney confirmed to be clear with an X-ray *in situ*. The renal pelvis is sewn up and the wound closed with drainage.

STONES IN THE URETER

Little dogs make the most noise

The pain of a stone in the ureter is excruciating. It comes on suddenly, in waves that make the patient roll and twist to get relief. Extravasation of urine into the retroperitoneal tissues causes vomiting and distension of the bowel that mimics intestinal obstruction. There may be tenderness over the loin and iliac fossa (Fig. 7.19). A trace of blood is often present in the urine.

Stones less than 5 mm in diameter will usually pass down the ureter on their own, at the expense of several bouts of pain that are usually relieved by diclofenac. If the stone is making steady progress and there is no infection, no operation is indicated. Infection calls for an immediate percutaneous nephrostomy.

When the stone is not making progress, is obviously too big, or remains stuck for several weeks, it is removed by ESWL. It can be broken up with an instrument introduced via the ureteroscope, but this carries a considerable risk of injury to the ureter and should be used only with the utmost caution.

The classical operation was open ureterolithotomy. Under general anaes-

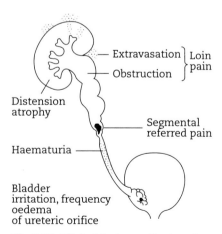

Fig. 7.19 Clinical features of a stone in the ureter.

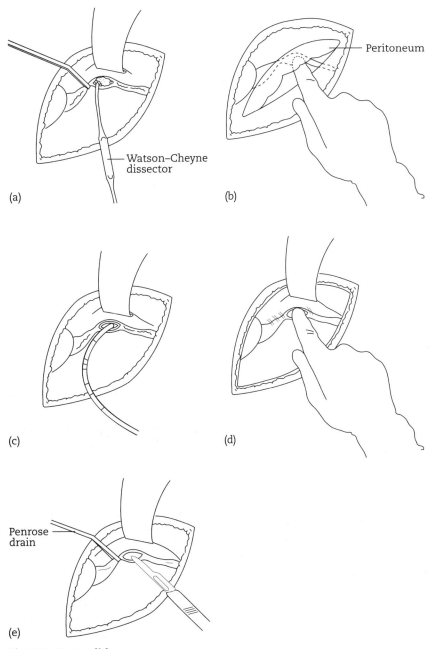

Fig. 7.20 Ureterolithotomy.

thetic a short incision was made over the appropriate part of the ureter, the peritoneum was reflected medially and the stone located with a finger. A short incision in the ureter allowed the stone to be prised out, and the wound was then closed with drainage. Unlike ureteroscopic operations, the incision in the ureter

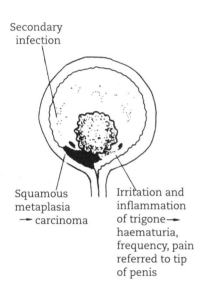

Fig. 7.21 Clinical features of a stone in the bladder.

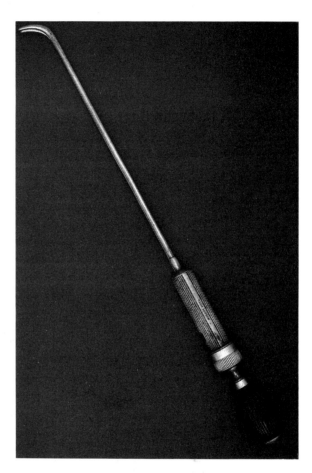

Fig. 7.22 Classical lithotrite.

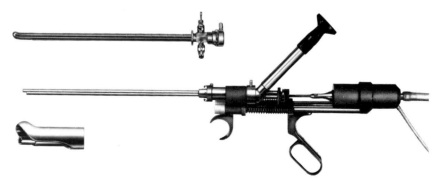

Fig. 7.23 Storz ultrasonic lithotriptor. Courtesy Rimmer Bros, UK Agents for Karl Storz.

always healed spontaneously, did not need to be sutured and was never followed by a stricture (Fig. 7.20).

STONES IN THE BLADDER

A stone that is small enough to pass down the ureter can usually get out of the bladder, and most ureteric stones pass without being noticed. Obstruction to the outflow of the bladder may trap the stones and today, in the West, bladder stones are seen only in elderly men with prostatic obstruction. In women, bladder stones are even more rare and have usually formed on a non-absorbable stitch.

The symptoms are those of outflow obstruction without pain or haematuria (Fig. 7.21), but sometimes pain is referred to the tip of the penis, and is made worse by exercise and is relieved by lying down.

Small bladder stones are seen through a resectoscope sheath, broken up with forceps and washed out. Larger ones are crushed with the classical lithotrite (Fig. 7.22), its modern visual counterpart (Fig. 7.23), the Swiss jack-hammer or the Q-switched laser.

In little boys, and in adults with very large stones that fill the bladder, a suprapubic lithotomy is safer. A short incision is made over the full bladder which is opened between stay sutures and the stone lifted out. The bladder is closed with an indwelling catheter that remains in place for 5–6 days.

FURTHER READING

Boyce WH, Pool CS, Meschan I, King JS (1958) Organic matrix of urinary calculi. *Acta Radiol* **50**: 544.

Embon OM, Rose GA, Rosenbaum T (1990) Chronic dehydration stone disease. *Br J Urol* **66**: 357.

Kamahira O, Ono Y, Katoh N, Yamada S, Mizutani K, Ohshima S (1996) Long-term stone recurrence rate after extracorporeal shock wave lithotripsy. *J Urol* **156**: 1267.

Marberger M, Fitzpatrick JM, Jenkins AD, Pak CYC (eds) *Stone Surgery*. Edinburgh, Churchill Livingstone.

Randall A (1937) The origin and growth of renal calculi. *Ann Surg* **105**: 1009.

Ryall RL (1994) Metabolic aspects of stone disease: graven images and pipe dreams. *Curr Op Urol* **4**: 223.

Swift-Joly J (1920) *Stone: Calculus Disease of the Urinary Organs*. London, Heinemann.

Tomson CRV (1995) Prevention of recurrent calcium stones: a rational approach. *Br J Urol* **76**: 419.

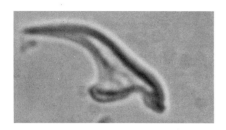

Neoplasms of the Kidney

EMBRYOMA (WILMS' TUMOUR)

Embryoma accounts for 10% of all childhood cancers and is seen in 1 : 13 000 children. There are two types, one inherited, the other not. The inherited group has an autosomal dominant with loss of genetic material on chromosome 11 and is associated with aniridia, hemihypertrophy, macroglossia, multicystic disease, neurofibromatosis and adult renal cell cancer.

In the first few months one particular subgroup has to be distinguished: it behaves almost as if it were benign — *mesoblastic nephroma*. It must be completely excised. One in 10 Wilms' tumours are bilateral.

There are two distinct pathological entities — favourable and unfavourable, according to the amount of undifferentiated tissue that is present and in practice the worst of this is usually rhabdomyosarcoma. Embryonal cancer spreads by direct invasion into the adjacent muscle and bowel: it may be carried in the bloodstream to the lungs. It erodes the renal pelvis relatively late, so that haematuria occurs late and carries a bad prognosis.

CLINICAL FEATURES

A big lump in a wasted baby

A mother bathing her baby notices a lump: this is the classical presentation (Fig. 8.1) but these tumours also cause pain and haematuria, as well as hypertension, fever, and a raised red or white cell count. The main differential diagnosis is from neuroblastoma. Ultrasound is the first investigation, and is followed by computed tomography (CT) scanning, even if this requires a general anaesthetic in a baby. In practice the differential diagnosis is from neuroblastoma (see p. 110), which usually has speckled calcification, and displaces the kidney downwards.

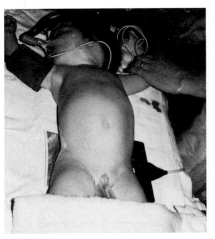

Fig. 8.1 Wilms' tumour—a big lump in a wasted baby.

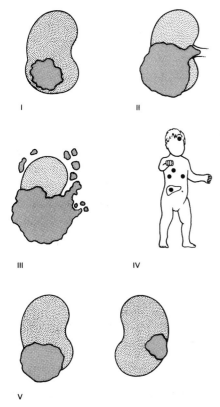

Fig. 8.2 Staging of Wilms' tumour.

Staging of Wilms' tumour (Fig. 8.2)

With a combination of radical surgery and chemotherapy one can expect more than 87% 4-year survival even in stage III with favourable histology, and this increases to over 96% in stage I disease. But to achieve these results expert management is called for and every child with a Wilms' tumour deserves to be referred to a specialized centre involved in trials of the latest protocols which regularly audits its results. It is not for the occasional surgeon in a small hospital.

One such protocol calls for a 5-day course of actinomycin D followed by laparotomy at which the renal vessels are tied before the tumour is handled, and the opposite kidney is carefully examined. The kidney is then removed radically, with a wide margin. Postoperatively vincristine is given.

Radiotherapy is not used in stage I tumours: it is always given in stage III, and its role in stage II is still under review.

RENAL CELL CANCER – GRAWITZ TUMOUR (HYPERNEPHROMA)

Grawitz tumour is a tumour of grandfathers (Fig. 8.3). It is very rare before puberty, and less common in females. It is associated with the von Hippel–Lindau syndrome where there are angiomas in the cerebellum and retina, and cysts in the liver and pancreas. It may be associated with cadmium pollution, and a growing number of new tumours are now being found by ultrasound scanning of patients on long-term renal dialysis.

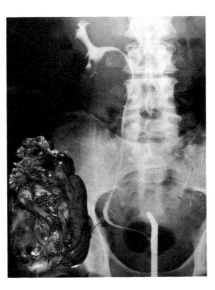

Fig. 8.3 Grawitz tumour.

PATHOLOGY

Many healthy adults have small 'adenomas' in their kidneys which arise from the renal tubule, are bright yellow, and resemble cancer in all histological respects. There is a nonsensical convention which calls them adenoma if they are less than 3 cm in diameter, and cancer if above 3 cm. But metastases occur from tumours which are less than 2 cm.

GRADE

Three grades are recognized according to frequency of mitosis. Flow cytometry has added nothing (Fig. 8.4).

STAGE

The International Union against Cancer (UICC) system (Fig. 8.5) is based on the findings on CT scanning and pathological examination of the excised specimen.

CLINICAL FEATURES

Most kidney cancers are detected incidentally when quite small because of ultrasound scanning done for some entirely unrelated reason. The classical symptoms of haematuria, pain, and a lump are all features of late, large cancers (Fig. 8.6). Haematuria means that the cancer has already eaten into the collecting system: pain means spread into the surrounding tissues, and if one can feel a lump it has to be very big indeed.

There is an interesting subgroup which present with features which can often be related to a specific chemical or hormone produced by the malignant renal cells:

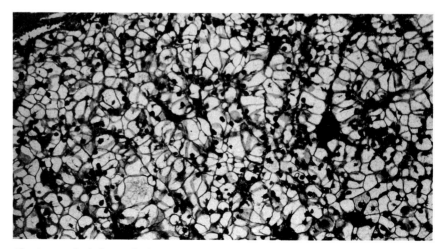

Fig. 8.4 Typical clear celled renal cell carcinoma of the kidney.

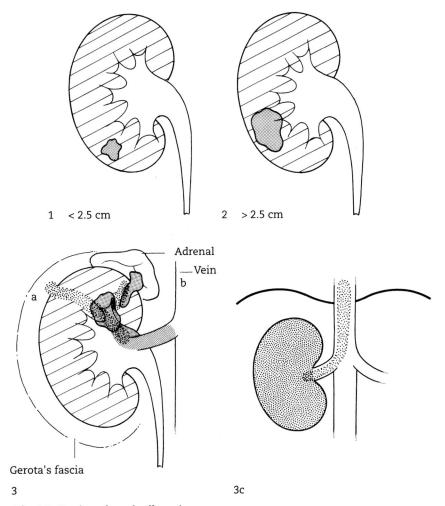

Fig. 8.5 Staging of renal cell carcinoma.

NEOPLASTIC HORMONE SYNDROMES IN RENAL CELL CANCER

Pyrogen	Loss of weight, pyrexia, night sweats, raised ESR
Erythropoietin	Erythrocytosis without increase in platelets
Marrow toxin?	Anaemia
Renin	Hypertension
Parathyroid hormone	Hypercalcaemia
Stauffer's factor	Hepatosplenomegaly
Glucagon	Diarrhoea, enteropathy
Tumour proteins	Glomerulonephritis
Amyloid	Amyloid in contralateral kidney
Unknown factor	Paraneoplastic motoneurone disease

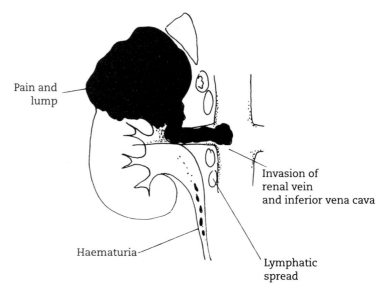

Fig. 8.6 Clinical features of renal cell carcinoma.

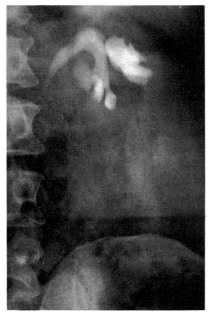

Fig. 8.7 IVU showing left renal pelvis grossly distorted by huge soft tissue mass arising from the lower pole.

DISTANT METASTASES

Finally many tumours are only detected when a distant metastasis is biopsied and the unmistakable histological picture of a renal cell cancer is found.

Investigations

Ultrasound shows a mass in the kidney which contains echoes. The intravenous urogram (IVU) and CT scan show a mass distorting the collecting system (Fig. 8.7) but may not be able to distinguish between a collection of cysts and cancer. With a very large tumour one needs to know whether the vena cava has been invaded: here magnetic resonance imaging (MRI) is more accurate than either CT or a cavogram (Fig. 8.8).

Treatment

SMALL TUMOURS

Many tumours are now being detected incidentally in the course of ultrasound and CT scanning when they are small enough to be removed leaving a safe clear margin of healthy tissue by partial nephrectomy.

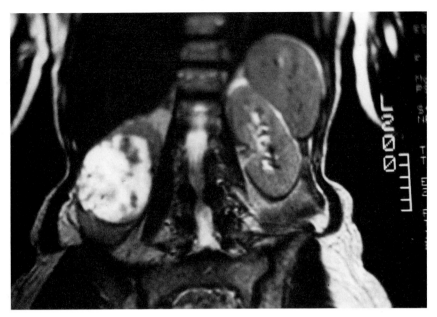

Fig. 8.8 MRI image showing renal cell carcinoma in right kidney.

PARTIAL NEPHRECTOMY

After exposing the kidney, the renal artery is secured. If it seems likely that the operation will be a long one, the kidney is packed in sterile ice-slush. The cancer is then removed with a clear margin (checked by frozen section). Every vessel is then suture ligated, and when complete haemostasis has been obtained the wound is closed.

LARGE TUMOURS—RADICAL NEPHRECTOMY

Through a generous incision either vertical or transverse—according to the build of the patient (Fig. 8.9)—the colon and duodenum are reflected from the front of the kidney (Fig. 8.10). The renal artery is ligated. Then the vein is divided between ligatures, and an intact block of tissue is then removed containing the kidney, all the surrounding fat inside Gerota's fascia, as well as the lymph nodes along the side of the aorta (on the left) or the vena cava (on the right).

When tumour is found growing into the inferior vena cava, after taping the cava, lumbar veins and opposite renal veins, the vena cava is opened without loss of blood, and the lump of tumour removed cleanly (Fig. 8.11).

When preoperative investigations have shown that the tumour has extended along the inferior vena cava into the heart, it has been shown that worthwhile survival can be obtained by removing the tumour extension, although this means very careful preliminary planning, and putting the patient on cardiac bypass.

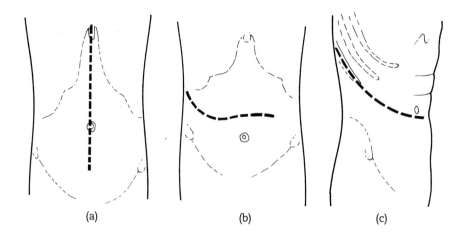

Fig. 8.9 Incisions for radical nephrectomy chosen according to the site and size of the tumour and the build of the patient.

(a)   (b)   (c)

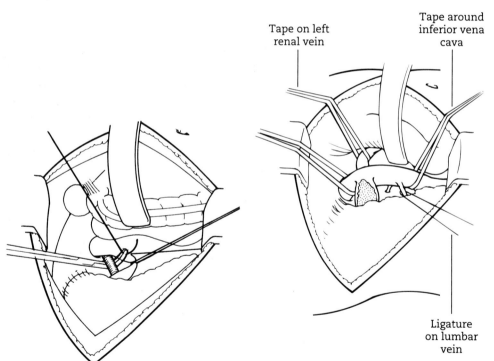

Fig. 8.10 The renal artery is ligated before mobilizing the mass.

Tape on left renal vein

Tape around inferior vena cava

Ligature on lumbar vein

Fig. 8.11 Extension of tumour into the inferior vena cava: the veins are all taped before opening the vena cava.

If the cancer is confined to the kidney, nephrectomy alone is followed by over 80% 5-year survival. The outlook is worse when the lymph nodes are involved or the fat and vena cava are invaded. Sometimes, miraculously, distant metastases go away once the primary tumour has been removed, suggesting that there might be a powerful natural immune system against renal cell cancer. Currently, attempts are being made to boost this immune mechanism with interleukin 2.

Radiotherapy and chemotherapy have so far proved useless.

Rare tumours that imitate renal cell cancer

Benign multilocular cysts imitate all the radiological, CT and ultrasonic features of the cystic form of a Grawitz cancer.

Angiomyolipoma is a tumour which is sometimes associated with tuberose sclerosis. Its content of fat gives it an unmistakable appearance in the CT scan. It can cause fatal retroperitoneal haemorrhage, and sometimes becomes malignant, so it should always be removed.

UROTHELIAL CANCER OF THE RENAL PELVIS AND URETER

The renal pelvis and ureter are lined with urothelium which is identical with that of the bladder, and gives rise to identical urothelial or transitional cell cancer. Urothelial cancer is seen in patients with recurrent bladder cancers and in the West is associated with smoking, analgesic and Balkan nephropathy, and Chinese slimming herbal remedies (see p. 70).

PATHOLOGY

Urothelial cancer in the upper tract, like that in the bladder, is classified in three grades, 1, 2 and 3: in addition metaplasia may be followed by squamous or adeno-carcinoma, both of which are usually very anaplastic. The tumours spread directly into the muscle of the pelvis and the renal parenchyma as well as into the surrounding fat. They can seed further down the urinary tract and they metastasize via lymph nodes rather than veins.

CLINICAL FEATURES

Haematuria is the most important symptoms: pain is late (see Fig. 12.23, p. 136).

INVESTIGATIONS

The IVU shows a filling defect (Fig. 8.12) which may be difficult to detect when the tumour is small. Malignant cells may be recognized on cytological examination of the urine in G2 and G3 tumours. The CT and ultrasound scans do not help. A retro-grade ureterogram gives a clearer picture of the filling defect, and a small brush may be used to acquire cells from the tumour for cytology. If the tumour is within reach of the ureteroscope it can be used to obtain a biopsy and allow the tumour to be coagulated with a laser (Fig. 8.13).

TREATMENT

The majority of these cancers are G3, multifocal, and have already invaded the muscle of the renal pelvis, so that the correct treatment is nephroureterectomy. However, when the tumour is well differentiated and still uninvasive, it is sometimes possible to perform a local resection. A working sheath is introduced as for percutaneous nephrolithotomy (see p. 82) and the tumour is coagulated with a

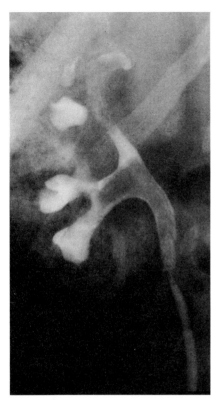

Fig. 8.12 Filling defects in the renal pelvis and calices from multifocal urothelial carcinoma of the right kidney. Courtesy of Dr W. Hately.

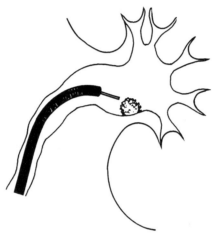

Fig. 8.13 Coagulation of a small tumour in the renal pelvis with the YAG laser through a flexible ureteroscope.

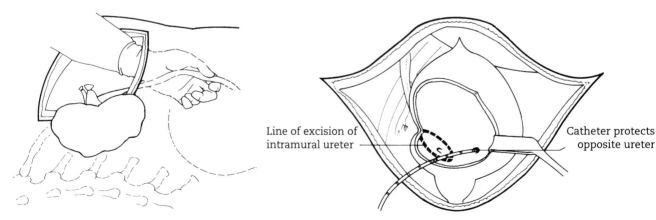

Line of excision of intramural ureter

Catheter protects opposite ureter

Fig. 8.14 Nephroureterectomy: (a) the kidney and ureter are mobilized; (b) the lower end of the ureter is removed with a cuff of trigone.

laser or diathermy. There is a risk that tumour cells may be implanted in the track so postoperative radiation is given. When local resection is not appropriate, the kidney may be approached through the 12th rib tip approach, as for pyelolithotomy (see p. 86), the pelvis is opened, and the tumour locally excised.

NEPHROURETERECTOMY

The kidney and ureter are removed *en bloc* (Fig. 8.14). If the ureter is left behind there is an almost inevitable chance of recurrence. In G3 tumours adjuvant radiotherapy is often given before the nephroureterectomy, or combination chemotherapy given afterwards.

FURTHER READING

Coppes MJ, Williams BRG (1994) The molecular genetics of Wilms' tumor. *J Nat Cancer Inst* **68**: 429.

Guinan PD, Vogelzang NJ, Fremgen AM *et al.* (1995) Renal cell carcinoma: tumor size, stage and survival. *J Urol* **153**: 901 (review).

Lanigan D (1995) Prognostic factors in renal cell carcinoma. *Br J Urol* **75**: 565 (review).

Pritchard J, Imeson J, Barnes J *et al.* (1995) Results of the UK children's cancer study group first Wilms' tumor study. *J Clin Oncol* **13**: 124.

Ritchey ML (1996) Primary nephrectomy for Wilms' tumor: approach of the National Wilms' Tumor Study Group. *Urology* **47**: 787.

Streem SB (1995) Percutaneous management of upper tract transitional cell carcinoma. *Urol Clin N Am* **22.1**: 221.

Taneja SS, Pierce W, Figlin R, Belldegrun A (1995) Immunotherapy for renal cell carcinoma: the era of interleukin-2 based treatment. *Urology* **45**: 911.

Vanherweghem JL, Tielemans C, Simon J, Depierreux M (1995) Chinese herbs nephropathy and renal pelvic carcinoma. *Nephrol Dial Transplant* **10**: 270.

Yao M, Shuin T (1995) Familial renal cell carcinoma: review of recent molecular genetics. *Int J Urol* **2**: 61.

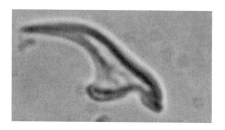

Vascular Disorders of the Kidney and Hypertension

ARTERIAL INFARCTION

Since the branches of the renal artery do not anastomose with each other if one of them is blocked its territory becomes infarcted. This is sometimes seen with mural thrombi following cardiac infarction. The patient has loin pain and haematuria, and urograms show atrophy of a segment of the kidney. If the main renal artery is blocked the entire parenchyma atrophies but the pelvis and collecting systems are not affected (Fig. 9.1).

VENOUS THROMBOSIS

The veins of the kidney intercommunicate freely with each other and with the veins in the surrounding fat so that even when the main renal vein is completely blocked recovery is usually complete (Fig. 9.2). Renal vein thrombosis is sometimes seen in children who are ill and dehydrated. They have pain and swelling in the loin, with profuse haematuria. A urogram may show no contrast on that side but in spite of this, recovery may be complete. In adults renal vein thrombosis may occur if intravenous contrast medium is given to a patient with amyloid.

ANEURYSM OF THE RENAL ARTERY

Aneurysms of the renal artery may be saccular or fusiform, and may involve the main segmental branches as well as the main artery. The wall is often calcified (Fig. 9.3). On clinical examination a bruit can be heard over the kidney. The diagnosis depends on good selective angiography (see p. 20).

TREATMENT

The risk of spontaneous rupture in a saccular aneurysm increases with size. Those that are less than 1 cm in diameter can safely be kept under observation, but those

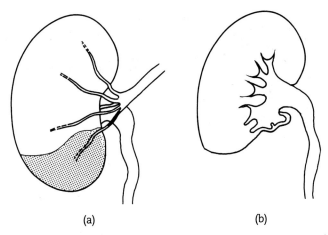

(a)   (b)

Fig. 9.1 Embolism in a segmental artery leads to infarction and atrophy of an entire segment.

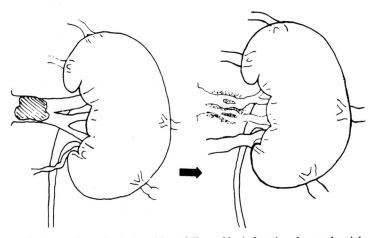

Fig. 9.2 Blockage of renal vein is seldom followed by infarction due to the rich collateral venous circulation.

over 2 cm should be operated on. Fusiform aneurysms may be associated with patchy narrowing of branches of the renal artery causing hypertension, and may require reconstruction.

ARTERIOVENOUS ANEURYSMS

Most of these follow trauma, including taking a renal biopsy. The shunting effect may give rise to heart failure. A similar kind of arteriovenous fistula is seen in some types of renal cell cancer. Nephrectomy is usually necessary.

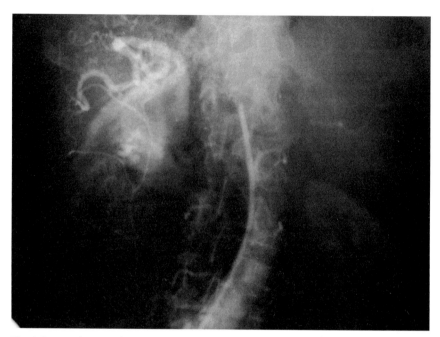

Fig. 9.3 Arteriogram showing aneurysm of right renal artery.

RENAL HYPERTENSION

The juxtaglomerular apparatus (see p. 33) continually monitors the pressure in the glomerular arteriole (Fig. 9.4). When the pressure is lowered, it secretes renin, an enzyme which splits one of the α_2-globulins in serum (angiotensinogen) to release angiotensin I. This is at first inactive, but on reaching the lungs is converted into angiotensin II, which has two powerful pharmacological effects: (i) it constricts peripheral arteries; and (ii) it stimulates the outermost layer of the adrenal cortex to secrete aldosterone which makes the distal renal tubules conserve sodium and water and increase the blood volume.

This renin–angiotensin mechanism can be triggered by a whole range of disorders of the kidney, including scarring from whatever cause, tuberculosis, cancer, polycystic disease, trauma and hydronephrosis. Its most striking form is seen when the main renal artery is stenosed.

INVESTIGATION

A renal cause should always be looked for in a young patient with hypertension because it can usually be corrected. An intravenous urogram (IVU) will reveal hydronephrosis or scarring. Dimercapto succinic acid (DMSA) isotope studies show an impaired blood flow, and angiography with digital vascular imaging will localize the stenosis in the renal artery (see p. 22).

Although one can measure plasma renin, it is easier to detect its action indi-

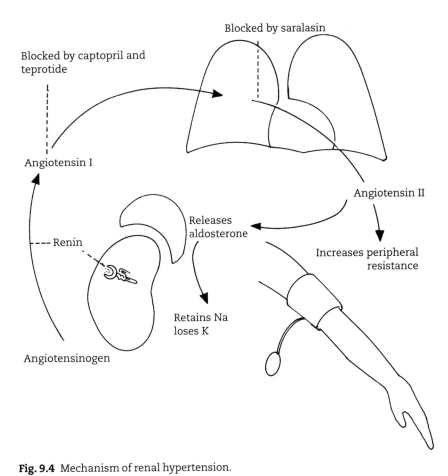

Blocked by captopril and
teprotide

Blocked by saralasin

Angiotensin I

Angiotensin II

Releases
aldosterone

Increases peripheral
resistance

Renin

Retains Na
loses K

Angiotensinogen

Fig. 9.4 Mechanism of renal hypertension.

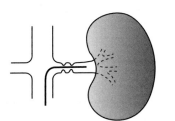

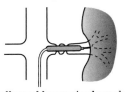

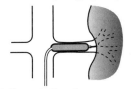

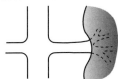

(a) Guide-wire passed through stenosis

(b) Followed by angioplasty balloon

(c) Balloon inflated

(d) Stenosis dilated

Fig. 9.5 Angioplasty.

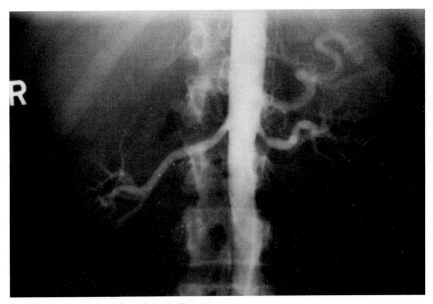

Fig. 9.6 Angiogram showing irregular beading of the left renal artery from
fibromuscular dysplasia.

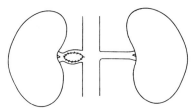

Patch on stenosed renal artery

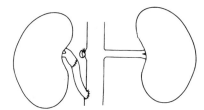

By-pass graft from aorta to distal healthy renal artery

Fig. 9.7 Patching or bypassing a renal artery stenosis.

rectly. Captopril and Teprotide block the release of angiotensin II in the lungs. Saralasin blocks the pharmacological effects of angiotensin II. If these substances lower the blood pressure one can assume that renin is responsible.

RENAL ARTERY STENOSIS

Atheroma may form a plaque at the origin of the main renal artery which can be treated by dilatation with a balloon catheter — angioplasty (Fig. 9.5). In dysplasia the artery is irregularly narrowed like a string of beads (Fig. 9.6), and may have to be bypassed with a graft, or enlarged by adding on a patch (Fig. 9.7).

When there is a small scarred kidney it is usually futile to try to deal with the narrowed artery, and better to perform nephrectomy, but when both kidneys are affected, one can obtain a useful improvement in renal function (or at least prevent further deterioration) by operating on the arteries.

FURTHER READING

Davidson RA, Wilcox CS (1992) Newer tests for the diagnosis of renovascular disease. *J Am Med Assoc* **268**: 3353.

Goldfarb DA, Novick AC (1994) The renin–angiotensin system: revised concepts and implications for renal function. *Urology* **43**: 572.

Lamawansa MD, Bell R, Kumar A, House AK (1995) Radiological predictors of response to renovascular reconstructive surgery. *Ann Roy Coll Surg Engl* **77**: 337.

Martin RS, Meacham PW, Ditesheim JA, Mulherin JL, Edwards WH (1989) Renal artery aneurysm: selective treatment for hypertension and prevention of rupture. *J Vasc Surg* **9**: 26.

Ramsay LE, Waller PC (1990) Blood pressure response to percutaneous transluminal angioplasty for renovascular hypertension: an overview of published series. *Br Med J* **300**: 569.

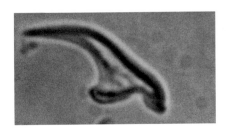

The Adrenal Gland

SURGICAL ANATOMY

Each adrenal gland lies just medial to the upper pole of the kidney. The arteries supplying the adrenal arise from the aorta, phrenic and renal arteries and are all quite small. The right adrenal vein drains into the vena cava: it is short and easily torn. The left adrenal vein enters the left renal vein (Fig. 10.1).

The adrenal gland is like a sandwich—the cortex—folded over a jam filling—the medulla. The cortex has three layers. The outer layer, the zona glomerulosa, secretes aldosterone. The middle layer, the zona fasciculata, secretes cortisol. The inner layer, zona reticularis, secretes androgens (Fig. 10.2). The medulla is made of sympathetic nerve endings and phaeochromocytes which secrete adrenaline and noradrenaline.

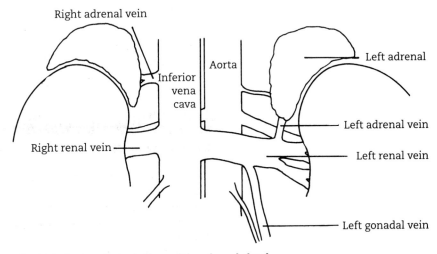

Fig. 10.1 Anatomical relations of the adrenal gland.

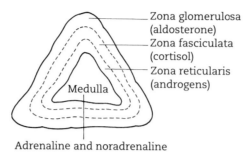

Zona glomerulosa
(aldosterone)
Zona fasciculata
(cortisol)
Zona reticularis
(androgens)
Medulla
Adrenaline and noradrenaline

Fig. 10.2 The folded sandwich arrangement of the adrenal.

ADRENAL TUMOURS

Tumours can arise from any part of the adrenal, and may or may not secrete the appropriate hormone.

NON-FUNCTIONING TUMOURS OF THE ADRENAL

These are usually detected by accident in the course of an ultrasound or computed tomography (CT) scan. From time to time they present with metastases. Size is the usual, but rather oversimple guide to malignancy: i.e. tumours less than 3 cm diameter are probably benign, those over 6 cm diameter are probably malignant. Each case has to be considered on its merits and sometimes a biopsy is required.

ZONA GLOMERULOSA TUMOURS (CONN'S SYNDROME)

These may be single or multiple and may occur on both sides. They are usually benign. The secretion of aldosterone leads to retention of sodium causing hypertension, and loss of potassium causing weakness. The diagnosis is made by the combination of a low plasma [K], high aldosterone, and low renin level. It is confirmed by giving spironolactone which reverses the picture. The patient can often be controlled with spironolactone but the side effects, e.g. enlargement of the breasts, indigestion and impotence, may be unbearable and the patient may prefer an operation. The adrenals are exposed through two 12th rib tip incisions. If a single adenoma is found the entire adrenal is removed: if both adrenals are involved with multiple adenomas, both are removed, and adrenal replacement given afterwards.

ZONA FASCICULATA TUMOURS (CUSHING'S SYNDROME)

The excess of cortisol gives the patient a buffalo hump at the back of the neck, hirsutes, a red face, subcutaneous haemorrhages, cutaneous striae, hypertension, diabetes and osteoporosis which may lead to pathological fractures (Fig. 10.3).

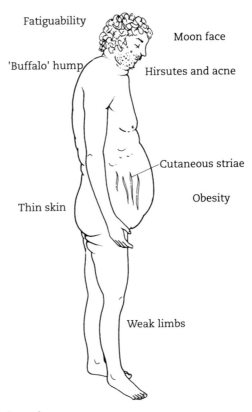

Fig. 10.3 Cushing's syndrome.

There may be a single cortisol-secreting tumour, or there may be bilateral hyperplasia which is sometimes caused by a basophil adenoma of the pituitary which is secreting adrenocorticotrophic hormone (ACTH). Very rarely the ACTH may be secreted by another tumour, e.g. carcinoma of the bronchus.

The diagnosis of Cushing's syndrome is made by measuring the urinary metabolites of cortisol, the 17-hydroxycorticosteroids. If due to ACTH stimulation, an intravenous dose of ACTH will increase these: if there is a primary adrenal tumour, a dose of dexamethasone will lower them.

If a CT scan reveals a primary adrenal tumour it is removed. If there is hyperplasia of both adrenals, a pituitary tumour must be excluded, and if none is found, then both adrenals are removed, and adrenal replacement given afterwards.

ZONA RETICULARIS TUMOURS: VIRILIZATION

Isolated tumours causing virilization are rare but an excess of androgens is often secreted by malignant adrenal tumours that are also producing cortisol. In children this causes increased growth, hirsutes, enlarged genitalia, a deep voice and in

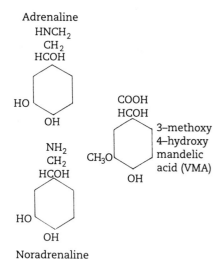

Adrenaline

Noradrenaline

Fig. 10.4 Adrenaline, noradrenaline and VMA.

girls, precocious menstruation. In adults there may be acne, hirsutes and disturbance of menstruation.

TUMOURS OF THE ADRENAL MEDULLA: PHAEOCHROMOCYTOMA

Phaeochromocytoma may occur in association with inherited disorders such as the multiple endocrine neoplasia type II and von Hippel–Lindau disease (see p. 93). They arise either in the adrenal medulla or on the aorta at the origin of the inferior mesenteric artery, and very rarely, in the bladder. The excess of adrenaline and noradrenaline causes paroxysms of hypertension with headache, sweating, flushing, tremor and pain in the chest.

DIAGNOSIS

A 24-h specimen of urine is acidified with hydrochloric acid, and measured for adrenaline, noradrenaline, and their metabolic end product, vanillylmandelic acid (VMA) (Fig. 10.4). During this test the patient avoids anything containing vanilla, e.g. bananas, chocolate and coffee. Although these tumours are so vascular that they show up with an angiogram, today they are located with a CT scan.

TREATMENT

The tumour must be removed. About 10% are malignant. To protect the patient from a sudden surge of catecholamines, phenoxybenzamine is given to block the α-receptors and propanolol to block the β-receptors. Even though these have been blocked, the tumour is handled as little as possible until the veins have all been ligated, at which moment the anaesthetist must be ready to deal with a fall in blood pressure. How the tumour is approached depends on its position: tumours near the adrenal are reached through a 12th rib tip incision; those near the inferior mesenteric artery through a midline laparotomy.

NEUROBLASTOMA

These are malignant tumours arising from nerve cell elements. They occur in toddlers, frequently with widespread metastases. The most common site of origin of the primary is in the region of the adrenal, but they can arise anywhere. They grow to an enormous size, and displace the kidney downwards. They must be distinguished from Wilms' tumours (see p. 92). Occasionally they secrete catecholamines and elevated levels of VMA are found in the urine. They are treated in specialized children's hospitals by a combination of surgery and chemotherapy.

FURTHER READING

Donohue JP (1988) Diagnosis and management of adrenal tumors. In: Skinner DG, Lieskovsky G (eds) *Diagnosis and Management of Genitourinary Cancer*. Philadelphia, WB Saunders, pp. 372–89.

Duckett JW, Koop CE (1977) Neuroblastoma. *Urol Clin N Am* **4**: 285.

Neville AM, O'Hare MJ (1979) Aspects of structure function and pathology. In: James VHT (ed.) *The Adrenal Gland*, vol. 2. New York, Raven Press, pp. 52–5.

Neumann JPH, Berger DP, Sigmund G *et al.* (1995) Phaeochromocytomas, multiple endocrine neoplasia type 2, and von Hippel–Lindau disease. *New Engl J Med* **329**: 1531.

Weiss LM (1984) Comparative histologic study of 43 metastasizing and non-metastasizing adrenocortical tumors. *Am J Surg Pathol* **8**: 163.

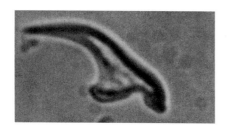

Renal Failure

ACUTE RENAL FAILURE

The causes of acute renal failure fall into three main categories which often occur together (Fig. 11.1).

1 Poor renal perfusion. Poor renal perfusion occurs in haemorrhage, trauma, burns, severe diarrhoea and vomiting, septicaemic shock and coronary thrombosis.

2 Renal tubular poisoning. Substances known to poison the renal tubules include mercury, phenol, carbon tetrachloride, glycol, and the toxin produced by *Clostridium welchii*.

3 Renal tubular blockage. Tubules may be blocked by (i) myoglobin when skeletal muscles have been crushed during injury; (ii) haemoglobin after mismatched transfusion or the transurethral resection (TUR) syndrome; (iii) porphyrins; (iv) bilirubin in severe jaundice; (v) crystals of sulphonamide if an incorrect dose is given; or (vi) crystals of uric acid during the massive protein catabolism that occurs when a tumour is responding to chemotherapy.

PATHOLOGY

The kidney is swollen, and the blood is usually shunted from cortex to medulla so that the medulla is congested and the cortex pale. The debris that clogs up the tubules resembles necrosis—hence the term acute tubular necrosis, which is misleading because the condition may be reversible, especially when mainly caused by underperfusion. If the cause cannot be reversed, then the cortex does indeed die, and a line of calcification may appear at the edge of the dead tissue (Fig. 11.2).

CLINICAL FEATURES

The cause of the acute renal failure will have its own particular symptoms, e.g. septicaemia or multiple trauma, but against this background three phases can be distinguished: prodromal, oliguria–anuria, and recovery.

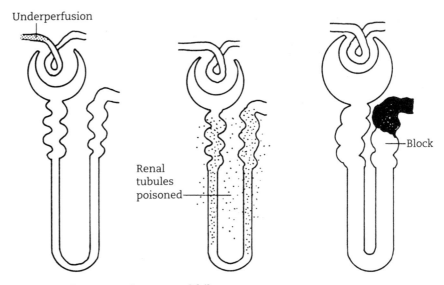

Underperfusion

Renal
tubules
poisoned

Block

Fig. 11.1 The causes of acute renal failure.

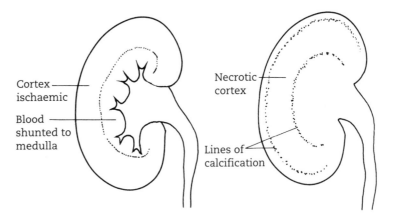

Cortex
ischaemic

Blood
shunted to
medulla

Necrotic
cortex

Lines of
calcification

Fig. 11.2 Necrosis of cortex with tramline calcification.

1   Prodromal phase. At first, while there is still some glomerular filtration, urine continues to form but is loaded with debris and granular casts.

2   Anuria or oliguria. After the prodromal phase comes a stage when there may be either no urine at all, or far too little to cope with the products of protein catabolism, e.g. urea, creatinine and phosphates. The blood urea, creatinine and potassium continue to rise, and any urine that is formed is pale and isotonic. The rate at which the waste products accumulate is accelerated when there is massive breakdown of tissue as a result of trauma or sepsis.

3   Recovery. At first the glomerular filtrate that starts to emerge is almost unprocessed by the sick tubules and soon the trickle is followed by a huge volume of dilute urine. During this phase the patient may have to be given many litres of fluid to prevent dehydration, and keep up with the massive losses of water and sodium.

MANAGEMENT

The aim of treatment is to keep the patient alive until the kidneys recover. This may take up to 6 weeks, during which time there is a continual breakdown of protein and accumulation of creatinine and potassium. During this period dialysis is performed, the choice of technique being determined by the underlying cause of the renal failure. Haemodialysis is used when there is intra-abdominal sepsis or when a very large amount of protein is being catabolized. In other cases peritoneal dialysis may be sufficient.

CHRONIC RENAL FAILURE

Sometimes renal function deteriorates very slowly, e.g. in polycystic disease (see p. 48), and the patient may be kept well on a diet low in protein. The restriction of protein to 40 g/day will keep down the plasma creatinine even when the clearance is only 20 ml/min. But eventually dialysis is called for, often because of intolerable symptoms.

CLINICAL FEATURES

1   Skin: patients develop itching and pigmentation of the skin.

2   Anaemia: want of erythropoietin leads to anaemia. Synthetic erythropoietin can correct this distressing feature.

3   Neuropathy, resulting from loss of myelin in peripheral nerves, causes weakness, numbness and paraesthesiae, especially in the feet.

4   Pericarditis may result in a pericardial effusion, and is a sign that the patient is being underdialysed.

5   Bone: the bowel becomes less sensitive to vitamin D, and so less calcium is absorbed. Growing bone is imperfectly calcified, forming osteoid rather than true bone — osteomalacia — which is weak and prone to fracture. At the same time phosphate accumulates and lowers the plasma [Ca], which stimulates the parathyroid to put out more parathyroid hormone (see p. 78). This causes calcium to be leached from the bones and deposited in soft tissues as heterotopic calcification which can cause stiffness of joints, especially in the middle ear, leading to deafness, as well as the rugger-jersey spine where stripes of decalcified bone alternate with bands of soft tissue calcification (Fig. 11.3).

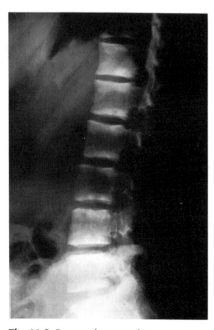

Fig. 11.3 Rugger-jersey spine.

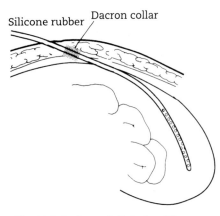

Silicone rubber   Dacron collar

Fig. 11.4 Peritoneal dialysis with Tenckhoff cannula.

DIALYSIS

CHRONIC AMBULANT PERITONEAL DIALYSIS

A silicone catheter is placed permanently in the pelvis (Fig. 11.4) and dialysis fluid is run in, left for several hours, and run out again after creatinine and products of catabolism have diffused into the fluid. Patients perform the instillation themselves. The main complication is, as might be expected, infection in the peritoneal cavity.

HAEMODIALYSIS

Blood from the patient is allowed to flow over a thin membrane separating it from dialysis fluid. There are a variety of devices, some of which are disposable and others used several times (Fig. 11.5). Unwanted products of catabolism diffuse out of the blood, while protein and red cells are retained. Access to the bloodstream is obtained with large-bore needles or a Scribner shunt (Fig. 11.6) tied into a paired artery and vein. For prolonged dialysis a peripheral artery is anastomosed to a vein to form an artificial arteriovenous fistula. Within a few weeks large varicose veins have formed into which the patient inserts needles enabling blood to run out through the machine and back again (Fig. 11.7). Repeated needling eventually leads to thrombosis of these fistulae and every year more ingenious techniques are devised to provide suitable vascular access for intermittent haemodialysis.

RENAL TRANSPLANTATION

The operation is in principle quite simple. A kidney from a living related donor or a cadaver is placed in one or other iliac fossa. The renal artery is anastomosed to the internal or external iliac artery, and the renal vein to the external iliac vein. The ureter is led through a tunnel into the bladder to prevent reflux (Fig. 11.8).

OBTAINING CADAVER KIDNEYS

It is always a waste when kidneys that could save two lives are allowed to decay in a dead patient. Relatives seldom refuse to give permission for kidneys to be used, and then usually only for religious reasons. The shortage of donors does not stem from the refusal of relatives, but from failure on the part of doctors and nurses to ask for permission, and a shortage of staff and facilities in intensive care units to keep patients on a ventilator after they are clearly brain-dead.

THE DONOR

Suitable donors must not have infection or cancer (except for some brain tumours). They should have extensive and irrecoverable brain damage, e.g. from severe head injury, intracranial haemorrhage, cardiac arrest or respiratory arrest.

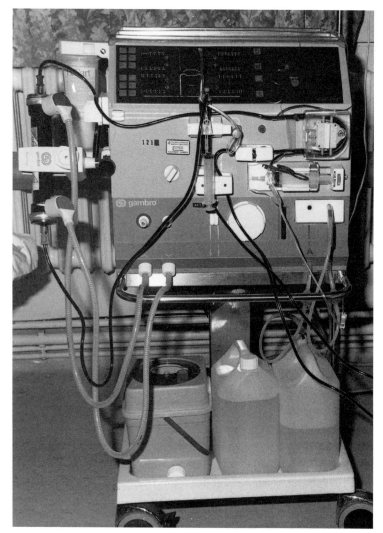

(a)

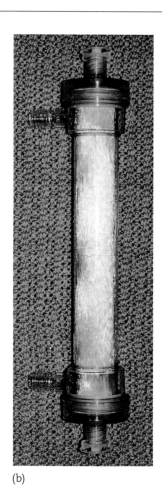

(b)

Fig. 11.5 (a) Artificial kidney and (b) disposable cartridge (courtesy of Dr Frank Marsh).

Such patients must be maintained on a ventilator. Strict tests are carried out to make sure that the brain damage is irreversible. Since not only kidneys but also other organs such as the heart, lungs and liver might be usable, the opportunity should never be lost to consider the possibility of using more than one organ.

REJECTION

A graft taken from one part of the body to another in the same person is not rejected, nor are grafts between identical twins. When a transplant from an unrelated person is performed for the first time, there is a latent period during which

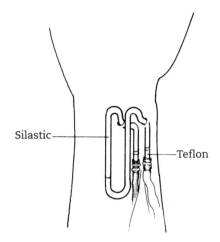

Silastic

Teflon

Fig. 11.6 Scribner shunt.

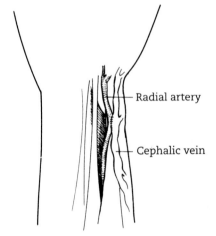

Radial artery

Cephalic vein

Fig. 11.7 Cimino fistula.

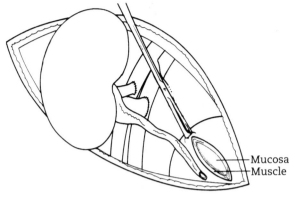

Mucosa
Muscle

Fig. 11.8 Renal transplant in right iliac fossa: the ureter is placed in a submucosal tunnel to prevent reflux.

the anastomoses heal and the kidney makes urine. Then, after about 10 days, lymphocytes in the regional lymph nodes enlarge, divide and migrate into the graft where they line the intima with immunoglobulin, which fixes complement and sets off the cascade of events that lead to thrombosis and infarction. This is the first set reaction.

A second graft from the same donor suffers the same fate, but much more quickly—second set reaction—because the patient is now sensitized to transplant antigens in the first graft. A graft from a different donor is handled by a first set reaction because the antigens that cause rejection are specific to each donor.

THE MAJOR HISTOCOMPATIBILITY SYSTEM

The transplant antigens (human lymphocyte antigens, HLA) are inherited on the sixth chromosome and expressed on the surface of every cell. Some are detected with serum antibodies (serum detected, SD). Others can only be detected in mixed lymphocyte culture where the host lymphocytes react to foreign lymphocytes by swelling up and undergoing division (lymphocyte activating determinants, LAD).

Rejection can only be prevented by getting an exact match between the HLA of host and donor but can be overcome by drugs which paralyse various components of the immune system. Three are in daily use: cyclosporin A, azathioprine and prednisolone. Cyclosporine is the most effective and least toxic: it works by preventing the formation of cytotoxic T-cells by the host. Azathioprine works in a similar way, but is more toxic. Steroids seem to complement azathioprine and may affect the function of lymphocytes. The prevention, recognition and treatment of rejection call for great skill and judgement.

HLA MATCHING

Because of the way homologous pairs of chromosomes are split at meiosis and

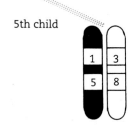

Fig. 11.9 Inheritance of the HLA genes.

transmitted by haploid gametes from parents to children, each child receives half its genetic programming from one parent and half from the other (Fig. 11.9). In any family with more than five children one pair must therefore always be identical with respect to their transplant antigens and if these children exchange kidneys there should be virtually no rejection. In fact this is not quite true because there are other, weaker antigens, and some immunosuppressive drugs are always needed unless the siblings are identical twins. However, a good HLA match can double the survival of transplants and for this reason kidneys are moved from one centre to another to ensure the optimum match.

LIVING RELATED DONORS

Transplants between siblings and between parents and children always share one complete set of transplant antigens, and generally do well. The donor kidney must be carefully investigated and proven to be healthy before it is used.

LIVING UNRELATED DONORS

The chance of finding a good HLA match in a living unrelated donor is always much smaller than in a relation, so much so that this is seldom done in the West, and is regarded as unethical and indeed unlawful if done as a commercial transaction.

REJECTION EPISODES

Hyperacute rejection

A recipient may unwittingly have been sensitized to antigens on the donor kidney so that as soon as blood enters the kidney there is an accelerated second set reaction: within minutes the kidney becomes thrombosed. These pre-existing cytotoxic antibodies can be detected by a cross-match, which is always performed prior to any transplant.

Accelerated rejection

This is a second set reaction and begins within 2 or 3 days of the transplant: it can respond to prompt diagnosis and intensive immunosuppressive treatment.

Acute rejection

Episodes of rejection may occur at any time after the transplant, but are most common in the first few weeks. The kidney becomes tender and swollen. The urine output diminishes, the diethylene triamine pentacetic acid (DTPA) clearance falls off (see p. 34) and Doppler studies show a diminished circulation. Fine-needle aspiration cytology from the graft shows blast cells and macrophages to be present. Larger doses of immunosuppressive agents, especially cyclosporin A, usually reverse the reaction. Acute rejection may come on many months after a transplant and may be precipitated by failure to take immunosuppressive medication or a blood transfusion.

Chronic rejection

There is a gradual failure of renal function which does not respond to immunosuppressive treatment. Eventually changes take place just like those of the end-stage kidney seen in other conditions (see p. 70). Eventually the kidney must be removed, and the patient is returned to dialysis and awaits another transplant.

PRESERVATION OF KIDNEYS FOR TRANSPLANTATION

An ice-cold solution — the Wisconsin University solution — which imitates the content of intracellular fluid, is used to wash out the donor kidney, which is placed in a pair of sterile plastic bags in a container surrounded by ice. Such a kidney will recover normal function even after 36 h of cold ischaemia time. What damages the kidney is the warm ischaemia time, i.e. the delay between cessation of perfusion of the kidney and its being cooled with preservative solution.

LONG-TERM RESULTS OF TRANSPLANTATION

There has been, and still is, a steady improvement in the results of renal transplantation so that more than 80% of cadaver kidneys are functioning at the end of a year. However, the difficulty of obtaining cadaver kidneys remains a major obstacle which will not be solved until every doctor and nurse concerned with a dying patient recognizes their responsibility, and until there is enough equipment and staff to provide ventilation for all brain-dead patients.

FURTHER READING

Breschia MJ, Cimino JE, Appel K et al. (1966) Chronic hemodialysis using venipuncture and a surgically created arteriovenous fistula. *New Engl J Med* **275**: 1089.

Gore SM, Hinds CJ, Rutherford AJ (1989) Organ donation from intensive care units in England. *Br Med J* **299**: 1193.

Jordan ML (1993) Immunosuppressive therapy and results of renal transplantation. *Curr Op Urol* **3**: 126.

Lumley JSP (1984) Vascular aspects of haemodialysis. *Br J Hosp Med* **32**: 244.

Morris PJ (ed.) (1988) *Kidney Transplantation: Principles and Practice.* 4th edition Philadelphia, WB Saunders.

Nicol DL (1995) Urologic aspects of renal transplantation. *Curr Op Urol* **5**: 86.

Odom NJ (1990) Organ donation 1. Management of the multiorgan donor. *Br Med J* **300**: 571.

Ploeg RJ, van Bockel JH, Langendijk PTH et al. (1992) Effect of preservation solution on results of cadaveric kidney transplantation. *Lancet* **340**: 129.

Scribner BH, Caner JEZ, Buri R, Quinton W (1960) The technique of continuous haemodialysis. *Trans Am Soc Artif Intern Organs* **6**: 88.

Smith R, Barnes AD, Bessey GS et al. (1983) *Cadaveric Organs for Transplantation: a Code of Practice including the Diagnosis of Brain Death.* London, DHSS.

Smithies MN, Cameron JS (1989) Can we predict outcome in acute renal failure? *Nephron* **51**: 297.

Tenckhoff H, Schechter H (1968) A bacteriologically safe peritoneal access device. *Trans Am Soc Artif Intern Organs* **14**: 181.

Wight C, Cohen B (1996) Shortage of organs for transplantation. *Br Med J* **312**: 989 (editorial).

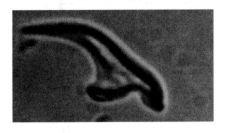

The Renal Pelvis and Ureter

ANATOMY

The ureters descend in front of the psoas muscle and the iliohypogastric and ileoinguinal nerves. Halfway down they are crossed in front by the vessels of the testis or ovary, and near the lower end by branches of the internal iliac artery and veins going to and from the uterus and bladder.

In women the ureter passes under a vascular band of fibrous tissue containing the uterine artery and veins (Fig. 12.1) where bleeding may occur during hysterectomy, and the ureter is easily injured in the course of efforts to secure haemostasis.

BLOOD SUPPLY OF THE URETER

The main blood supply of the ureter comes from the inferior segmental artery of the kidney (Fig. 12.2), which runs down the ureter, and is reinforced by unimportant small branches from the lumbar arteries. Towards the lower end it is joined by an ascending branch of the superior vesical artery. If the ureter is divided near the bladder this ascending branch is cut and the lower end of the ureter may be ischaemic.

NERVE SUPPLY OF THE URETER

Sensory nerves from the ureter follow a segmental pattern: the upper part, like the kidney, is supplied by T10, and pain is referred to the umbilicus. Lower down pain is referred to more caudal segments until pain from the lowest part of the ureter is referred to the vulva or tip of the penis (S3) (Fig. 12.3).

PERISTALSIS IN THE URETER

The ureter is lined by urothelium on a thin layer of submucosa (Fig. 12.4) outside

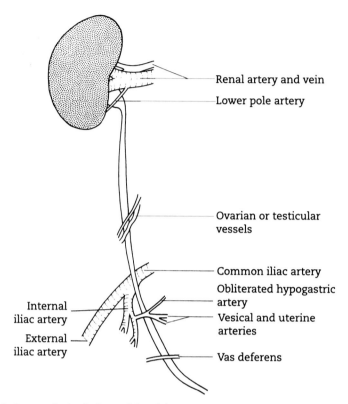

Fig. 12.1 Anatomical relations of the right ureter.

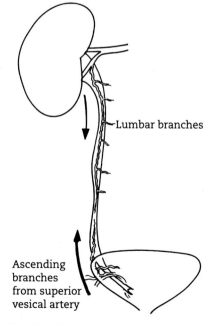

Fig. 12.2 Blood supply of the ureter.

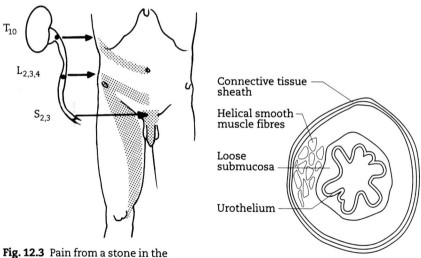

Fig. 12.3 Pain from a stone in the ureter is referred to relevant dermatome.

Fig. 12.4 Transverse section of the ureter.

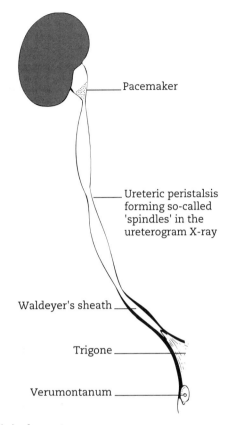

Fig. 12.5 Peristalsis in the ureter.

which the smooth muscle cells are connecting with each other so that excitation passes along the muscle without the need for nerves or ganglia (Fig. 12.5). Peristalsis in the ureter can be provoked by pinching or irritation. Thanks to this system the denervated transplanted ureter functions perfectly well.

Ureteric peristaltic waves speed up as more urine is formed until the point is reached when the walls of the ureter no longer come together and it functions as a drainpipe. To allow free movement of the ureter during peristalsis it is surrounded by a thin slippery sheath of connective tissue.

DIAGNOSIS OF OBSTRUCTION IN THE URETER

To distinguish between a ureter that is obstructed from one that is widened from some other reason, Whitaker's test is performed. A fine percutaneous nephrostomy tube is introduced into the renal pelvis (see p. 20) and contrast medium is run in at a rate known to be more than the maximum likely to be encountered during diuresis, e.g. 10 ml/min. If the pressure rises it means there must be obstruction downstream in the ureter (Fig. 12.6).

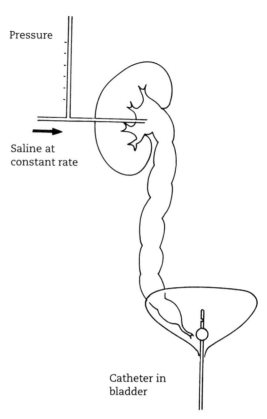

Fig. 12.6 Whitaker's test.

CONGENITAL ABNORMALITIES

The embryology of the ureter and some of the more important congenital abnormalities are described on p. 40. It may be helpful to be reminded of a few of them.

In duplex the ureteric bud branches early, and the ureter from the smaller upper half-kidney drains into the trigone caudal to that from the lower, larger half-kidney. In ectopic ureter the ureter from the upper half-kidney opens into the vagina downstream of the urethral sphincter and causes continual incontinence (Fig. 12.7). In ureterocele there is a balloon-like swelling where the ureter opens into the bladder, which may obstruct the ureter, allow a stone to form in its stagnant pool, or prolapse and obstruct the urethra. Most ureteroceles cause no trouble and need no treatment: the very large ones can be incised, but then there may be reflux requiring reimplantation (Fig. 12.8).

Reflux has been considered in relation to urinary infection (see p. 62). One of the less common conditions seen with duplex kidney is yo-yo reflux (see p. 42) where urine runs from the lower half-kidney to the upper one (Fig. 12.9).

Blind-ending duplex is another rare anomaly. One of the duplex ureters fails to rendezvous with its part of the metanephros and fails to induce a kidney. The result is a kind of ureteric 'diverticulum' which may harbour infection but usually needs no treatment at all.

Ureteric atresia has been noted in connection with dysplasia and congenital cysts of the kidney (see pp. 46 and 47).

Megaureter

This is a common and important entity in children which causes much confusion because it is so often assumed that when a dilated ureter is discovered in an

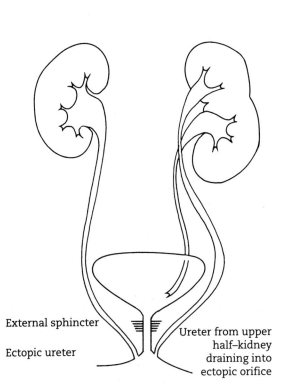

Fig. 12.7 If an ectopic duplex ureter opens downstream of the sphincter there is incontinence.

External sphincter

Ectopic ureter

Ureter from upper half–kidney draining into ectopic orifice

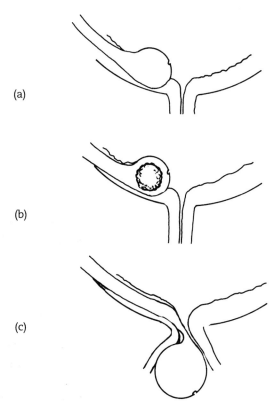

(a)

(b)

(c)

Fig. 12.8 Ureteroceles may (a) cause no trouble at all; (b) cause obstruction and possibly a stone; (c) prolapse into the urethra to cause acute retention of urine.

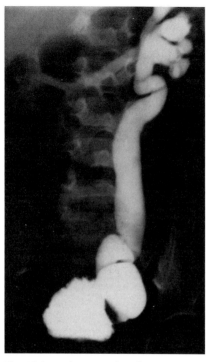

Fig. 12.9 Vesicoureteric reflux.

ultrasound scan or an intravenous urogram (IVU) there must necessarily be obstruction.

1   Reflux. Most megaureters are caused by reflux (Fig. 12.9) (see p. 62).

2   Congenital stenosis at the lower end of the ureter. A narrowing, from an unknown cause, occurs at the lower end of the ureter, giving rise to obstruction upstream (Fig. 12.10). Diagnosis may need a Whitaker's test.

3   Idiopathic. In a number of boys the ureters are found to be huge, but there is no reflux, and no narrowing at the lower end. The cause is a mystery. One plausible suggestion is that at some time in fetal life there was a posterior urethral valve (see p. 221) which gave rise to gross obstruction and dilatation of the ureters, and then the valve ruptured spontaneously, leaving the child with large ureters without any apparent reason for them.

The important message is that surgical interference will only improve matters when there is reflux or an obstruction.

PELVIURETERIC JUNCTION OBSTRUCTION

This is a common condition. There is a ring of fibrous tissue where the renal pelvis

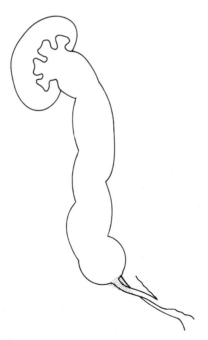

Fig. 12.10 Obstructed ureter caused by stenosis at the lower end.

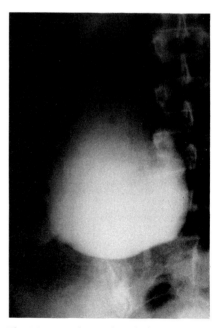

Fig. 12.11 Hydronephrosis from obstruction at the pelviureteric junction.

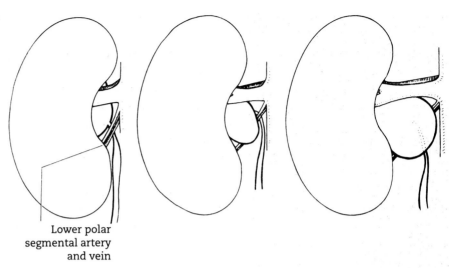

Lower polar
segmental artery
and vein

Fig. 12.12 The obstructed renal pelvis often bulges out between the two lower segmental arteries.

joins the ureter, of unknown cause. The renal pelvis and calices are obstructed and undergo dilatation—hydronephrosis (Fig. 12.11).

Hydronephrosis is often detected by ultrasound scanning in the fetus. Many of these show spontaneous cure during follow-up and surgical correction is only required if there is a deterioration in renal function, as judged by serial dimercapto succinic acid (DMSA) renography (see p. 36).

Hydronephrosis may be noted at any time in later life: at first its symptoms are often intermittent, so that pain occurs only when patients drink a lot, and because the pain follows a meal it is easy to misdiagnose a peptic ulcer.

The dilated renal pelvis bulges forwards between the two lower branches of the renal artery giving rise to the idea that an 'anomalous' renal artery is the cause of the obstruction (Fig. 12.12).

DIAGNOSIS
The difficulty in practice is to distinguish between a large baggy renal pelvis and one that is dilated because of obstruction. A diethylene triamine pentacetic acid (DTPA) renogram (see p. 34) is performed, and after a few minutes frusemide is given to cause a diuresis. If there is obstruction the isotope continues to accumulate in the renal pelvis: in a normal pelvis the isotope is washed away in the next few minutes (Fig. 12.13).

When the kidney is very distended it is sometimes difficult to know whether it

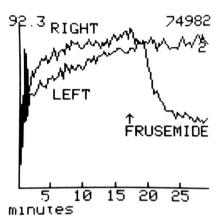

Fig. 12.13 DTPA renogram showing retention of isotope in the left kidney in spite of frusemide.

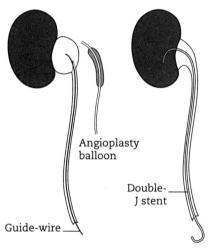

Fig. 12.14 Balloon pyeloplasty.

is worth trying to save it. A DMSA scan will show how much useful renal parenchyma there is.

MANAGEMENT

Patients found by chance to have a large renal pelvis, but no DTPA evidence of obstruction, can safely be kept under observation year after year. In those with obvious obstruction, or severe symptoms, then something needs to be done to overcome the obstruction.

Balloon dilatation

An angioplasty catheter is passed up the ureter over a guide-wire into the narrow segment and distended there. A double-J stent is left *in situ* for 10–14 days (Fig. 12.14).

Percutaneous ureterolysis

A working sheath is introduced into the renal pelvis as for percutaneous nephrolithotomy (see p. 82). Using a nephroscope, a guide-wire is passed down the ureter over which a knife is passed to incise the fibrous ring in the wall of the ureter. This is followed with a double-J stent which is left in position for about 6 weeks (Fig. 12.15).

Pyeloplasty

If these simple non-invasive methods are not feasible, or have been tried but without success, then a formal pyeloplasty is performed. First a ureterogram is made to define the length of the narrow segment of the ureter (see p. 18). Then the kidney is approached through an anterior transverse incision. The peritoneum is reflected to reveal the pelvis and ureter. The junction between ureter and pelvis is carefully dissected free, and a U-shaped flap of pelvis is let into the slit-open ureter as a gusset. The anastomosis is stented with a double-J splint or a nephrostomy for about 10 days (Fig. 12.16).

Retrocaval ureter

Very rarely the postcardinal veins of the embryo fail to become obliterated, and the ureter has to wind round behind the inferior vena cava. The intravenous urogram (IVU) appearance is unmistakable (Fig. 12.17). There is no need to meddle with the little bit of ureter behind the cava. The lower end is detached and anastomosed to the dilated upper part just as in any other hydronephrosis.

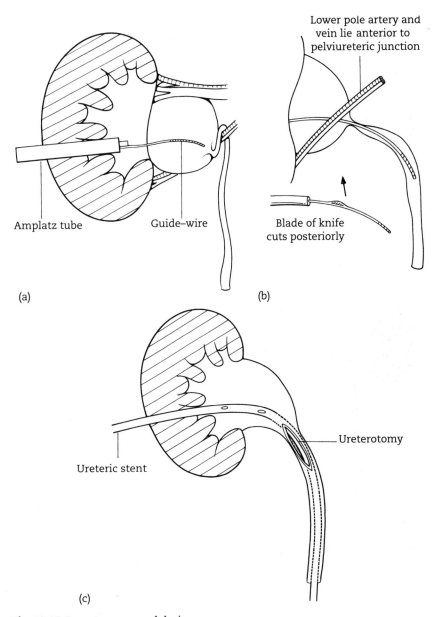

Fig. 12.15 Percutaneous pyelolysis.

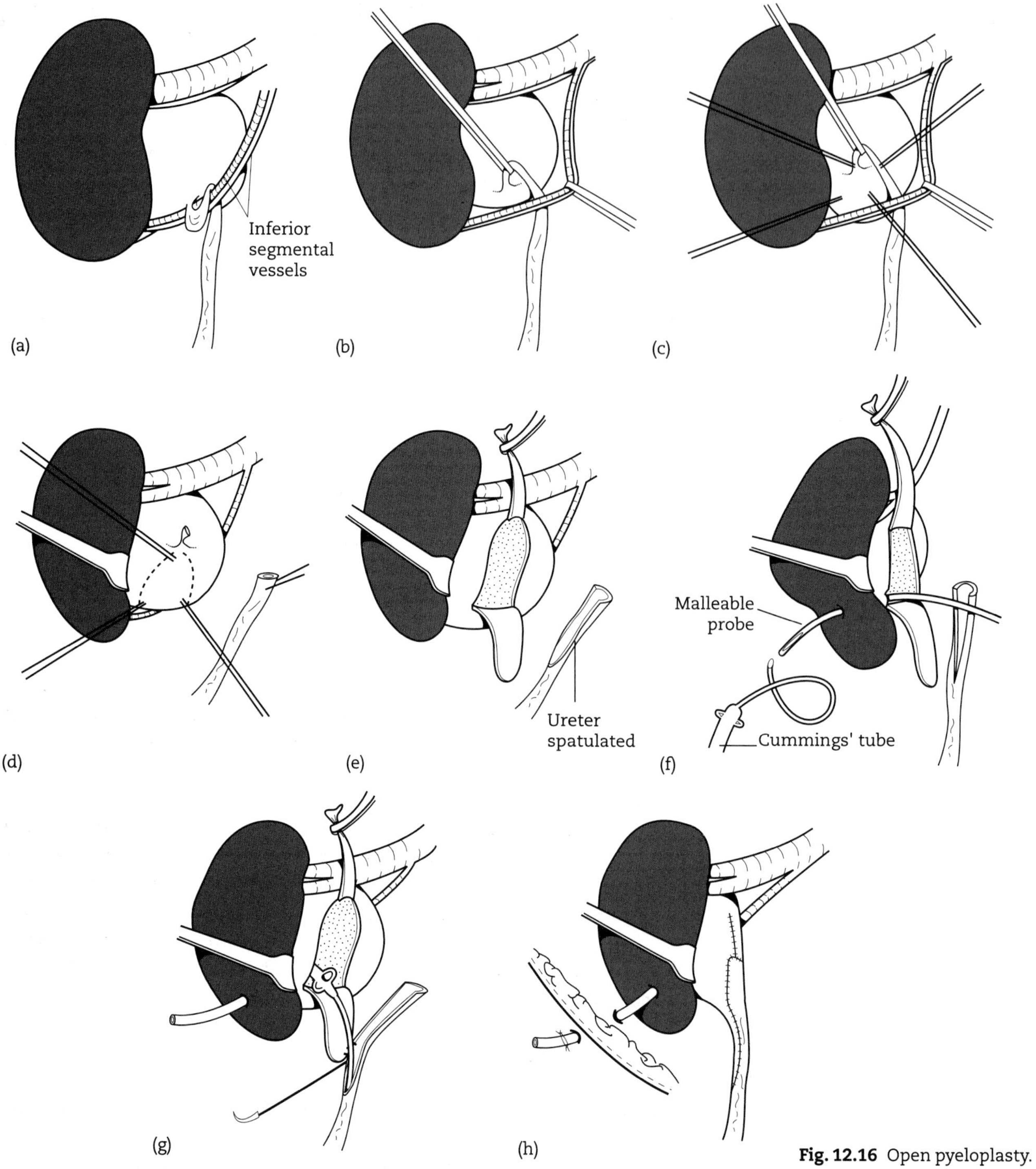

(a)

Inferior
segmental
vessels

(b)

(c)

(d)

(e)

Ureter
spatulated

(f)

Malleable
probe

Cummings' tube

(g)

(h)

Fig. 12.16 Open pyeloplasty.

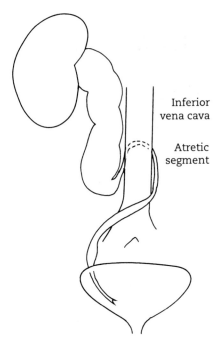

Inferior
vena cava

Atretic
segment

Fig. 12.17 Retrocaval ureter.

URETERIC INJURY

ACCIDENTAL TRAUMA

Closed injuries of the ureter are very rare. Open injuries caused by a knife or bullet are easily overlooked at the time the wound is explored, and may only be noticed afterwards when urine leaks from the wound.

IATROGENIC TRAUMA

The ureter is at risk in any operation in the pelvis, especially hysterectomy. The ureter is most prone to be injured where it is crossed by the uterine arteries and veins, which so often bleed profusely during the operation. It can also be caught higher up by a suture used to close the peritoneum. There are three distinct clinical scenarios.

Injury noticed at operation

If the injury is noticed at operation, and the ureter is healthy, it may be repaired by end-to-end anastomosis using non-absorbable sutures. The anastomosis should be protected by a suitable splint. Unfortunately the anastomosis may not heal owing to ischaemia in the lower part of the ureter (see p. 121).

Immediate postoperative symptoms

Pain in the loin and fever

More often the injury to the ureter is not noticed during the operation. The patient may have pain in the loin afterwards, and if the urine is infected, a fever. These are very important symptoms and demand an immediate IVU.

Anuria

If both ureters have been obstructed at the time of injury, the patient will be anuric. In practice the problem arises in just the kind of operation where there is likely to have been considerable loss of blood, and it is reasonable to think that shock has caused renal failure from underperfusion (see p. 112). Two things help: (i) in anuria from acute renal failure, there is nearly always *some* urine, however little, and it is full of granular casts; and (ii) when there is any doubt, an IVU should be done: if there is obstruction there will be a delayed nephrogram (see p. 17).

Late leak of urine

Far more often the pain in the loin has been put down to normal postoperative discomfort, and it is not for 7–10 days that fluid begins to escape from the vagina, by which time the patient has often gone home. The first and most urgent task is to confirm that the fluid which is leaking is urine. This is easy: have it sent to the

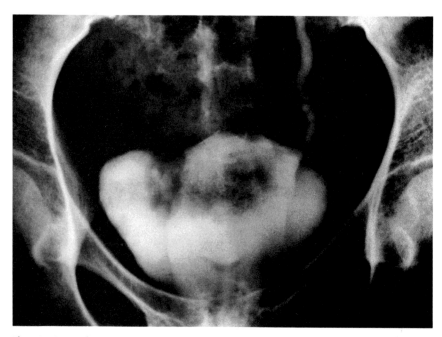

Fig. 12.18 IVU in ureterovaginal fistula following hysterectomy: contrast medium outlines the vagina. The ureter is a little obstructed.

laboratory for an urgent creatinine measurement. If the creatinine is greater than that in the blood the fluid just has to be urine.

The second step is to get an IVU. This will usually show some obstruction, and occasionally will show extravasation of the contrast into the vagina or soft tissues (Fig. 12.18).

Forget the traditional arcane ritual of putting a series of swabs into the vagina or methylene blue into the bladder. These only confuse the issue and waste time. Forget also the tradition that one must delay intervention for 40 days and 40 nights (or some such nonsense). The sooner the diagnosis is confirmed and the injured ureter is repaired the better (and the easier to do).

URETEROGRAM

A bulb-ended catheter is placed in the ureter and contrast injected. This will show extravasation or a block. It ought to be done on the other side as well since the injury is all too often bilateral (Fig. 12.19).

REPAIR OF THE URETER

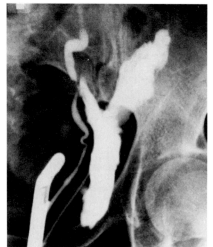

Fig. 12.19 Retrograde ureterogram showing contrast leaking out from the ureter. Courtesy of Mr J.C.Smith.

The previous incision is reopened. The ureter is traced down to the site of injury, which is usually a confused puddle of pus, urine and granulation tissue. The ureter

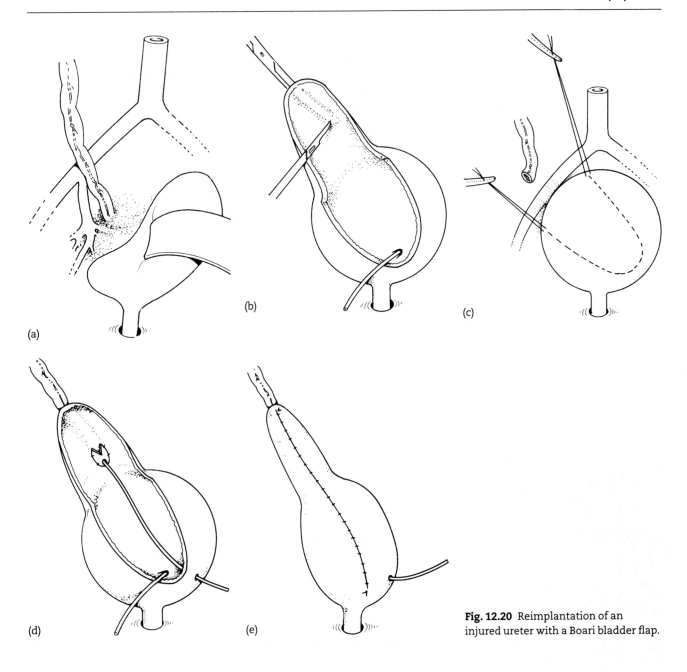

(a)

(b)

(c)

(d)

(e)

Fig. 12.20 Reimplantation of an injured ureter with a Boari bladder flap.

is divided where it is healthy, and implanted into a U-shaped (Boari) flap made from the wall of the bladder, with a tunnel to prevent reflux (Fig. 12.20).

INFLAMMATION OF THE URETER

ACUTE
Acute ureteritis may explain much of the pain in the groin which patients so often describe during acute urinary infection. It is rarely investigated or documented, and always recovers completely with time and antibiotics.

CHRONIC

Ureteritis cystica
Following a prolonged urinary infection the IVU or ureterogram may show multiple rounded filling defects in the ureter and renal pelvis. These are caused by a par-

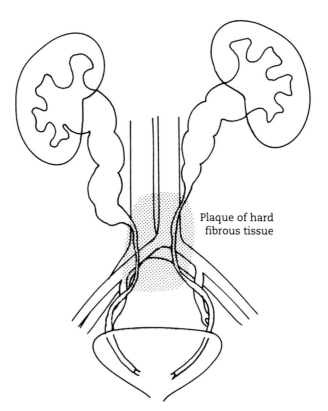

Plaque of hard fibrous tissue

Fig. 12.21 Retroperitoneal fibrosis.

ticular kind of chronic inflammation of the urothelium—ureteritis cystica—where little nests of urothelium get buried and swell up to form tiny cysts. It resolves completely in time.

Tuberculosis
The ureter is often involved in tuberculosis (see p. 68).

Bilharziasis
The wall of the ureter is always involved in bilharziasis (see p. 158). Pairs of *Schistosoma* flukes nest in the submucosal veins and lay eggs which provoke chronic inflammation, turning the ureter into a stiff, inert tube which is dilated, obstructed and often calcified.

Retroperitoneal fibrosis
Metastatic cancer, usually arising from the colon, may convert the retroperitoneal

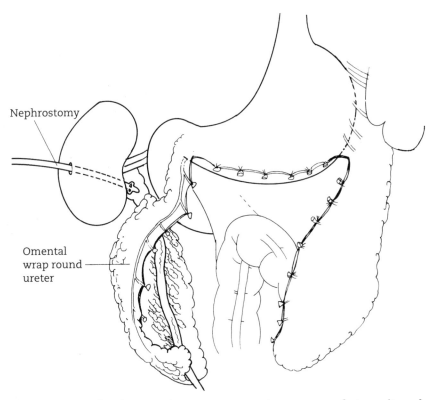

Fig. 12.22 Wrapping the ureter in omentum prevents recurrence of retroperitoneal fibrosis.

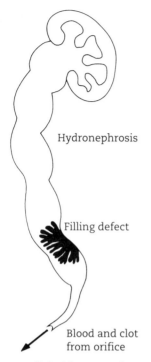

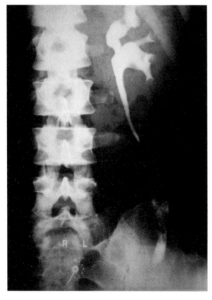

Fig. 12.23 Clinical features of a carcinoma of the ureter.

Fig. 12.24 IVU showing filling defect in the lower ureter caused by carcinoma. Courtesy of Dr W. Hately.

tissue into a hard plaque inside which the ureters cannot wriggle freely. Something similar is rarely seen in association with inflammation of the bowel in Crohn's disease or ulcerative colitis. But the most interesting of these types has no known cause, and is therefore called idiopathic retroperitoneal fibrosis.

These patients have backache, fever, loss of weight, an elevated sedimentation rate and hypertension. The ureter is encased in a stiff plaque of fibrous tissue, and cannot writhe sideways or up and down, and so becomes obstructed, even though it is easy to pass a catheter up and down. By the time the diagnosis is made the patient is often severely uraemic. The same plaque of fibrous tissue encases the vena cava and aorta, and may extend up into the porta hepatis and mediastinum (Fig. 12.21).

The first step is to relieve the obstruction with percutaneous nephrostomy (see p. 19). Once the patient has recovered from the uraemia, it is necessary to distinguish this from the other types of fibrosis listed above. Prednisolone has occasionally been reported to produce rapid and complete resolution of the obstruction, but more often the improvement is slow and incomplete. A more certain method is to free the ureters from the surrounding fibrous tissue, and wrap them in omentum to stop it coming back (Fig. 12.22).

All these patients must be very carefully followed up because they usually develop other complications of hypertension.

CARCINOMA OF THE URETER

Since the ureter is lined with urothelium it can form all the types of transitional cell cancer that are seen in the renal pelvis and bladder (see pp. 99 and 162). They present with haematuria, or pain from obstruction to the ureter (Fig. 12.23).

DIAGNOSIS
The diagnosis is suggested by the IVU, and confirmed by a ureterogram (Fig. 12.24). Malignant cells may be found in the urine on cytology if the tumour is G2 or G3.

TREATMENT
Single G1 tumours can occasionally be removed locally, but unfortunately they are usually multiple. G3 tumours have a very bad prognosis, and have often invaded through the wall of the ureter by the time they are detected, so that in addition to nephroureterectomy, adjuvant radiotherapy or chemotherapy is usually necessary.

STONES IN THE URETER

See p. 88.

FURTHER READING

Anderson JC, Hynes W (1949) Retrocaval ureter: case diagnosed preoperatively and treated successfully by plastic operation. *Br J Urol* **21**: 209.

Blandy JP, Fowler CG (1996) Idiopathic hydronephrosis. In: Blandy JP (ed.) *Urology*, 2nd edn. Oxford, Blackwell Science, pp. 107–20.

Gottschalk CW (1960) Observations on the intrarenal pressure. In: Quinn EL, Kass EH (eds) *Biology of Pyelonephritis*, Boston, Little, Brown, p. 131.

Huang A, Low RK, White R deV (1995) Nephrostomy tract tumor seeding following percutaneous manipulation of a ureteral carcinoma. *J Urol* **153**: 1041.

Ormond JK (1949) Bilateral ureteral obstruction due to envelopment and compression by one inflammatory process. *J Urol* **59**: 1072.

Struthers NW, Contaninou CE (1992) Ureteric physiology. *Curr Op Urol* **2**: 310.

Thompson AS, Dabhoiwala NF, Verbeek FJ, Lamers WH (1994) The functional anatomy of the ureterovesical junction. *Br J Urol* **73**: 284.

Tiptaft RC, Costello AJ, Paris AMI, Blandy JP (1982) The long-term follow-up of idiopathic retroperitoneal fibrosis. *Br J Urol* **54**: 620.

Whitaker RH, Buxton-Thomas M (1984) A comparison of pressure flow studies and renography in equivocal upper urinary tract obstruction. *J Urol* **131**: 446.

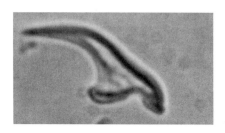

The Bladder: Structure and Function

SURGICAL ANATOMY

In children the bladder is an abdominal organ, easily felt and aspirated. In adults it cannot be felt unless it is distended because it lies deep in the symphysis. Above, the dome of the bladder is covered by peritoneum, against which lie loops of small bowel and sigmoid colon. A long tail of urachus tethers the dome of the bladder to the umbilicus: this is the vestige of the fetal allantois.

As the bladder becomes distended it rises, not always in the midline, and it may bulge out into the inguinal canal to form the 'bladder ears' so often seen in cystograms in normal children. In adults the bladder is just medial to the neck of an inguinal or femoral hernia.

Posteriorly the bladder is separated from the rectum by the fascia of Denonvilliers which is made of the two fused layers of peritoneum. This forms a remarkable biological barrier: it prevents carcinoma of the bladder or prostate spreading into the rectum (Fig. 13.1).

In the male the bladder rests on the prostate gland, below which is the levator ani muscle. In females the bladder rests on the anterior wall of the vagina (Fig. 13.2).

The fibres of the detrusor muscle of the bladder are not arranged in layers (as in the bowel) but run criss-cross, like a basket, each fibre passing from outer to inner layers and back again. Outside the bladder there is no capsule, as in other viscera: its muscle lies against fat, connective tissue and a plexus of large veins.

The detrusor muscle is lined by a thin layer of submucosa on which lies the waterproof urothelium (Fig. 13.3).

BLOOD SUPPLY

The arteries come from branches of the internal iliac artery of which the largest, the superior vesical artery, crosses in front of the ureter (Fig. 13.4). The veins of the bladder drain into the internal iliac veins, but in addition, a second 'backstairs' system drains into the marrow of the pelvic bones, femora and vertebral bodies,

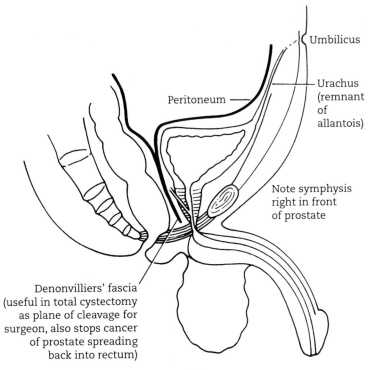

Fig. 13.1 Surgical anatomy of the male bladder.

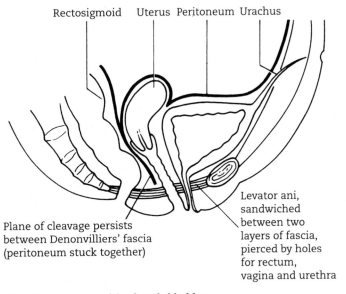

Fig. 13.2 Surgical anatomy of the female bladder.

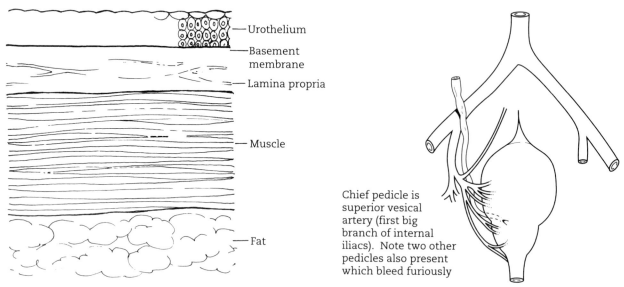

Fig. 13.3 Diagram of section through wall of bladder.

Fig. 13.4 Blood supply of the bladder.

so that any increase in intra-abdominal pressure forces blood from the bladder into the marrow, hence metastases from cancer of the prostate and bladder are often found there.

There is a rich network of lymphatics in the deeper layers of the detrusor muscle, which drains into the lymph nodes of the pelvis. Like the veins, there are also direct communications with the bone marrow of the pelvis, vertebrae and femora.

NERVES OF THE BLADDER

Afferent impulses from the bladder pass up in the pelvic parasympathetic nerves— nervi erigentes — to the S2, S3 segments of the spinal cord. Sensation of pain is also conveyed in sympathetic fibres which run via the presacral plexus and lumbar sympathetic ganglia to reach surprisingly high levels in the spinal cord: hence to block all pain from the bladder a spinal anaesthetic must reach as high as T6. The fibres of both sets of autonomic nerves reach the bladder along the arterial branches (Fig. 13.5).

The S2, S3 segments of the spinal cord lie in the conus medullaris at the level of T12, L1, which is just where the back is most often injured in traffic or industrial accidents.

From the S2, S3 segments efferent motor impulses go to the bladder along three sets of nerves:

1 parasympathetic fibres to ganglia in the wall of the detrusor muscle causing it to contract;

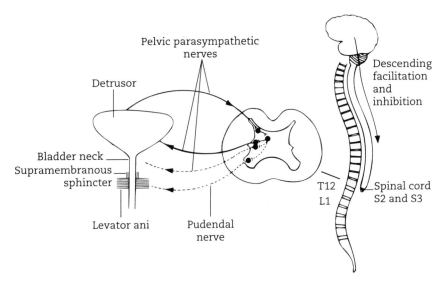

Fig. 13.5 Nerve supply of the bladder.

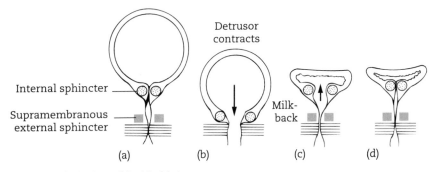

Fig. 13.6 Emptying of the bladder.

2 sympathetic fibres to the supramembranous sphincter and the neck of the bladder;

3 somatic myelinated fibres in the pudendal nerve supply the striated muscle of the levator ani.

MICTURITION

Filling of the bladder stimulates stretch receptors which send impulses up the parasympathetic afferent fibres. The reflex arc in the S2, S3 segments sends impulses back to the detrusor along parasympathetic fibres causing it to contract, and at the same time, inhibits the efferent sympathetic impulses going to the bladder neck and supramembranous sphincter, as well as those going in the myelinated fibres of the pudendal nerve to the levator ani and pelvic floor.

When the bladder has been emptied out, first the pelvic floor contracts, then the supramembranous sphincter milks back urine from the prostatic urethra into the bladder, and finally the bladder neck is closed (Fig. 13.6). Like all reflexes, that for micturition is modified by influences from higher up in the nervous system which may either facilitate or inhibit the reflex arc. We all are aware that on occasions the urge to empty an overdistended bladder drives all other thoughts from consciousness, and that anxiety or fright may bring on an urge to urinate.

URODYNAMICS

CYSTOMETRY

Through a fine catheter, water is slowly run into the bladder while its pressure (Pves) is continually recorded through a second catheter, either alongside the first in the urethra, or introduced through a small needle suprapubically (Fig. 13.7). A third catheter is placed inside the rectum to measure intra-abdominal pressure (Pabd), and a computer subtracts this from the intravesical measurement to give the true detrusor pressure (Pdet) (Fig. 13.8).

The measurements are made while the bladder is filled, and while the patient

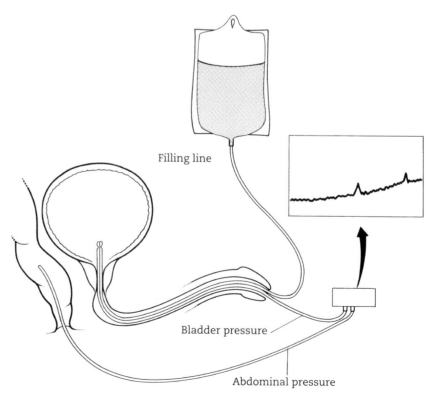

Filling line

Bladder pressure

Abdominal pressure

Fig. 13.7 Cystometry.

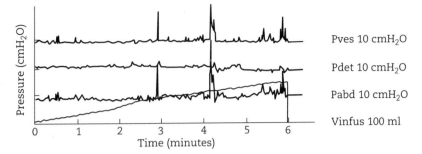

Fig. 13.8 Cystometrogram.

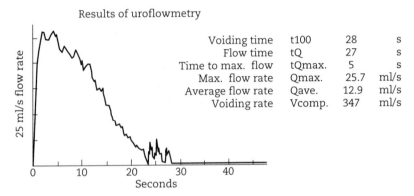

Fig. 13.9 Normal uroflow measurement.

passes urine into an electronic flow meter, a device that automatically records the flow rate (Qmax) and the volume of urine that has been collected (Vcomp) (Fig. 13.9).

VOIDING CYSTOMETROGRAM

These measurements are often combined with a video X-ray recording of the cystogram, by using dilute contrast medium instead of water. Study of the recording allows one to see the bladder neck opening and closing, and to note any reflux of urine up the ureters.

ELECTROMYOGRAPHY

In exceptional cases the activity of the striated muscle of the levator ani can be recorded from small needle electrodes inserted into the muscle. This is not a routine investigation and calls for considerable experience in its use and interpretation. At rest there is normally a constant level of activity in the levator ani, which, when the electromyogram is connected to a loudspeaker, sounds like a constant buzz. While the bladder is emptying and the impulses down the pudendal nerve are inhibited, there should be silence (Fig. 13.10).

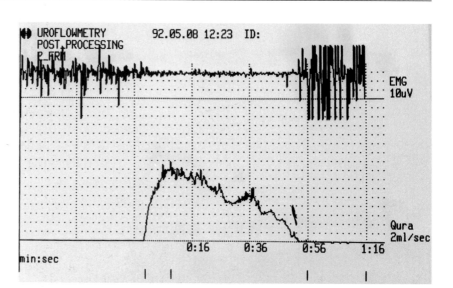

Fig. 13.10 Electromyogram from external sphincter during voiding (courtesy of Dr C Fowler).

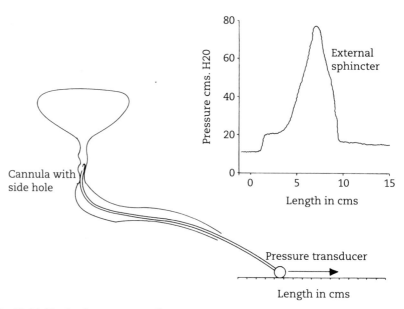

Fig. 13.11 Urethral pressure profile.

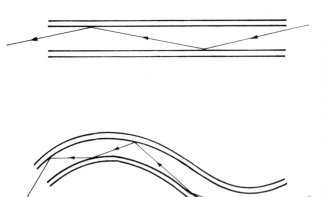

Fig. 13.12 Total internal reflection along a glass fibre.

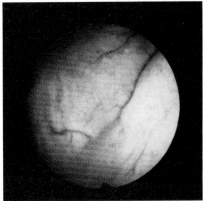

Fig. 13.13 Image obtained through flexible cystoscope.

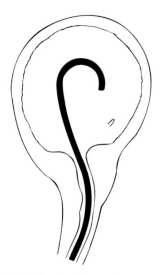

Fig. 13.14 The flexible cystoscope can give a view of the trigone and bladder neck.

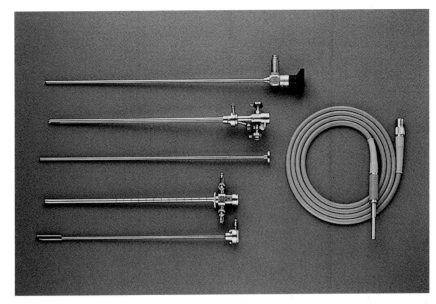

Fig. 13.15 Variety of instruments used in modern cystoscopy.

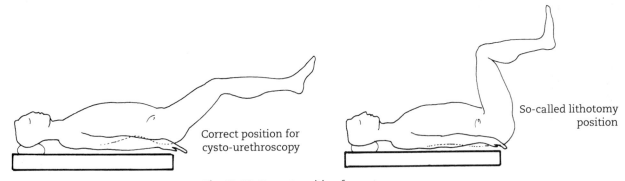

Correct position for cysto-urethroscopy

So-called lithotomy position

Fig. 13.16 Correct position for cystoscopy.

URETHRAL PRESSURE PROFILE

The pressure inside the lumen of the urethra can be measured with a catheter that is withdrawn at a constant rate along the urethra. The pressure is drawn on a graph which measures the distance along the urethra, giving the urethral pressure profile. This is not a routine investigation, but is of help in some cases of incontinence (Fig. 13.11).

CYSTOSCOPY

FLEXIBLE CYSTOSCOPY

Fine glass fibres are flexible. If made of completely clear optical glass, and coated with glass of a different refractive index, all the light entering one end will leave the other (Fig. 13.12). A large number of these fibres are wound on a wheel, glued at one spot, and cut through. The result is a fibre-optic cable which can be introduced into any orifice of the body, and will transmit an image in a series of tiny dots like ground glass (Fig. 13.13).

The modern flexible cystoscope has channels for irrigation, for light, and for passing flexible instruments such as biopsy forceps, laser fibres or a diathermy electrode. Passing the cystoscope is painless. It is gently advanced along the urethra under vision as water is slowly run in. After examining the urethra, sphincter, prostatic urethra and bladder neck, the inside of the bladder is carefully inspected. By bending the cystoscope back on itself the bladder neck and prostate can be viewed from inside (Fig. 13.14).

RIGID CYSTOSCOPE

The image seen through the rigid cystoscope is much more clear than that of the flexible instrument, and the instrument channel allows a large variety of gadgets to be used inside the bladder (Fig. 13.15). Biopsies can be taken, tumours resected, stones crushed, ureters catheterized and examined. It is less comfortable for the patient than the flexible cystoscopy, and for some of these manoeuvres a general or spinal anaesthetic is required. The patient is placed in the cystoscopy position (Fig. 13.16).

FURTHER READING

Barrington FJF (1914) The nervous mechanism of micturition. *Q J Exp Physiol* **8**: 33.
Mundy AR, Stephenson TP, Wein AJ (1984) *Urodynamics, Principles, Practice and Application.* Edinburgh, Churchill Livingstone.
Narayan P, Koney B, Aslam K *et al.* (1995) Neuroanatomy of the external urethral sphincter: implications for urinary continence during radical prostatic surgery. *J Urol* **153**: 337.
Woodburne RT (1960) Structure and function of the urinary bladder. *J Urol* **84**: 79.

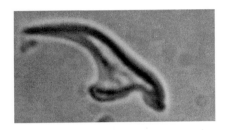

The Bladder: Congenital Abnormalities and Trauma

EMBRYOLOGY

The embryology of the bladder is outlined on p. 41. During the complicated processes in which the fetal hindgut, the cloaca, curls round so that its tip becomes the urachus, and the urogenital septum comes down to separate the future bladder from the rectum, bringing with it the mesonephric ducts which sprout the ureters, there are many opportunities for things to go wrong, and a large number of congenital abnormalities are seen in practice.

AGENESIS

The cloaca may not form at all: both ureters are obstructed, and the condition is not compatible with survival.

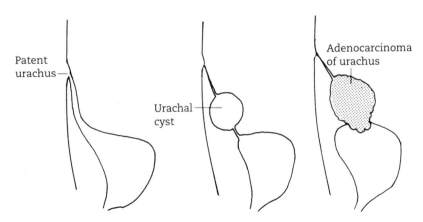

Fig. 14.1 Disorders of the persistent urachus.

DUPLICATION

Very rarely the bladder is divided by a septum either in the midline or lying transversely.

PATENT URACHUS

If there is obstruction at the neck of the bladder or the urethra the urachus may remain patent and leak urine at the umbilicus. Cysts may form in the remnant of the urachus and may become infected in later life, and because the urachus is a remnant of the hindgut, and is lined with bowel epithelium, it can give rise to an adenocarcinoma. This presents with haematuria, and on cystoscopy a small red lump like a cherry is seen at the apex of the bladder which is much smaller than the mass which can be felt outside (Fig. 14.1).

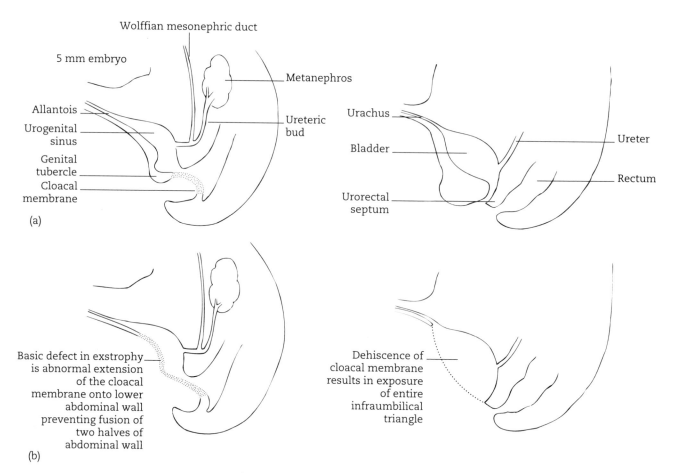

Fig. 14.2 The role of the cloacal membrane in the cause of exstrophy.

EXSTROPHY

In early fetal life the cloacal membrane may extend up to the umbilicus, and prevent the ingrowth of the future abdominal wall (Fig. 14.2). Normally the cloacal membrane dissolves only at the future anus, vagina and urethra. In exstrophy it exposes tissue below the umbilicus which varies from a dorsal cleft in the penis— epispadias—to the entire cloaca. In the most common variety, the bladder opens like a flat red patch on the abdomen onto which the ureters discharge urine. It is often accompanied by prolapse of the rectum, undescended testes, and wide separation of the symphysis pubis (Fig. 14.3).

Untreated, the condition is miserable. The child is continually soaked in urine. The exposed urothelium is always irritated, painful and inflamed, and eventually glandular metaplasia may go on to develop adenocarcinoma. All this can be prevented.

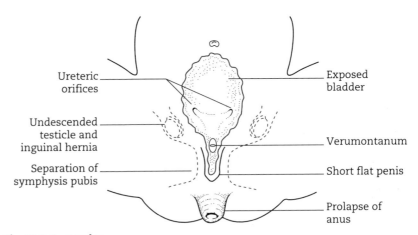

Fig. 14.3 Exstrophy.

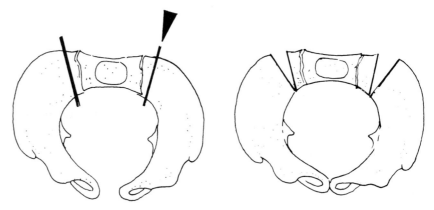

Fig. 14.4 Iliac osteotomy to assist closure of exstrophy.

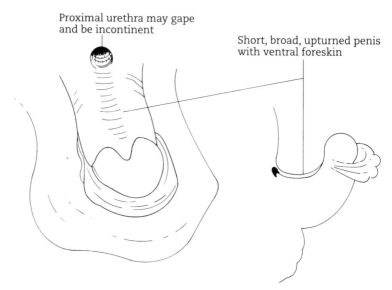

Proximal urethra may gape
and be incontinent

Short, broad, upturned penis
with ventral foreskin

Fig. 14.5 Epispadias.

Firstly, it is important to reassure the distraught parents that all will be well. Secondly, transfer the baby to a specialist paediatric unit where the operation to close the bladder is performed as soon as possible after birth. The bladder is mobilized, sewn into a sphere, and the abdominal wall closed over it. The sacro-iliac joints may be divided to allow the pelvis to be closed like an oyster (Fig. 14.4). Additional operations will be required later to reconstruct the bladder neck to restore continence, to reconstruct the penis, and to bring down the testicles. Eventually these children can grow up to lead a normal life: the boys have a normal sex life, and the girls can have children.

EPISPADIAS

In this minor version of exstrophy the urethra opens on the proximal end of the dorsum of a short flat penis which curves upwards (Fig. 14.5). This can also be completely refashioned in expert hands: first a new urethra is formed, and later the bladder neck may have to be reconstructed to restore continence.

TRAUMA

Open and penetrating injuries

The bladder may be injured in any penetrating abdominal injury. It is closed with absorbable sutures and a catheter is left in for about a week. The same man-

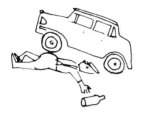

Fig. 14.6 Closed injury to the bladder.

agement is used when the bladder is opened in the course of some abdominal operation. The outcome is a perfectly functioning bladder.

One new type of penetrating injury has recently become of importance: people with a patch of small intestine added on to the bladder to increase its capacity or cure detrusor instability often have to catheterize themselves, and from time to time the catheter may perforate the bladder. The clinical features are those of a delayed perforation (see below).

Closed injury: intraperitoneal rupture

The typical patient is run over while he lies drunk and with a distended bladder (Fig. 14.6). The bladder bursts and a large volume of urine enters the peritoneal cavity but it is dilute and does not at first cause any chemical irritation. Only after several hours does the patient become ill (see below).

DIAGNOSIS

Paracentesis
If there is some reason to think there may be other intra-abdominal injuries, a four-quadrant tap is performed. If it shows blood, laparotomy or laparoscopy is performed and if a tear is found in the bladder, it is repaired with absorbable sutures and a catheter left in the bladder.

Cystogram
A cystogram may show contrast leaking into the peritoneal cavity, but only if the bladder is fully distended.

Cystoscopy
A flexible cystoscopy will show the tear.

TREATMENT
If there is no evidence of peritonitis an indwelling catheter can be left in the bladder for about a week, and then tested with a cystogram to show that the tear has healed.

Delayed perforation

After coagulation of a small recurrent cancer in the bladder, the necrotic wall of the bladder may give way about a week later, and allow urine to leak into the peritoneal cavity. Typically there is very little pain, and there are almost no abnormal physical signs at first, but after a few hours the abdomen becomes distended and the bowel sounds can no longer be heard. Paracentesis will yield evil smelling fluid.

If detected early, the condition is relieved by keeping the bladder emptied with a catheter, but if there is any doubt, or if the patient's condition is not improving, laparotomy, evacuation of the fluid, and repair of the lacerated bladder is the safest course.

FURTHER READING

Abrahamson J (1961) Double bladder and related anomalies: clinical and embryological aspects and a case report. *Br J Urol* **33**: 195.

Blandy JP, Badenoch DF, Fowler CG, Jenkins BJ, Thomas NWM (1991) Early repair of iatrogenic injury to the ureter or bladder following gynecological surgery. *J Urol* **146**: 761.

Canning DA (1996) Bladder exstrophy: the case for primary bladder reconstruction. *Urology* **48**: 831.

Hochberg E, Stone NN (1993) Bladder rupture associated with pelvic fracture due to blunt trauma. *Urology* **41**: 531.

Iuchtman M, Rahav S, Zer M, Mogilner J, Siplovich L (1993) Management of urachal anomalies in children and adults. *Urology* **42**: 426.

Lee JY, Cass AS (1993) Lower urinary and genital tract trauma. *Curr Op Urol* **3**: 194.

Marshall VF, Muecke EC (1962) Variations in exstrophy of the bladder. *J Urol* **88**: 766.

Mollard P, Mouriquand PDE, Buttin X (1994) Urinary continence after reconstruction of classical bladder exstrophy (73 cases). *Br J Urol* **73**: 298.

Salvatierra O, Rigdon WO, Norris DM, Brady TW (1969) Vietnam experience in 252 urological war injuries. *J Urol* **101**: 615.

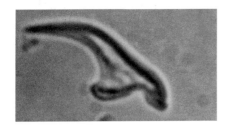

The Bladder: Inflammation

ACUTE CYSTITIS

In males acute cystitis usually signifies an important underlying disorder that needs thorough investigation. In females acute cystitis is very common. In either gender the cause is usually an intestinal pathogen such as *Escherichia coli*, *Klebsiella*, *Proteus mirabilis* or *Streptococcus faecalis*. Recurrent infections may be due to the original strain of microorganism or a new one. Rarer causes of cystitis include Herpes *virus hominis*, *Chlamydia* and *Neisseria gonorrhoeae*. Cystitis may occur when something has lowered the local resistance, e.g. diabetes mellitus, or minor local trauma as may occur in sexual intercourse.

Chemicals may cause inflammation without any microorganisms: examples include chemical cystitis from detergents added to bath-water, deodorants sprayed on the vulva, or chemicals such as cyclophosphamide that are secreted in the urine.

Whether caused by bacteria or a chemical, the clinical features of acute cystitis are those of inflammation anywhere else: the urothelium lining the bladder becomes red, oedematous and painful. The afferent arc of the micturition reflex is stimulated and the patient needs to empty her bladder before it is normally full. Pus and urothelial cells make the urine cloudy, while bacterial conversion of urea into ammonia gives it a fishy smell. There may be haematuria (Fig. 15.1).

The cystoscopic appearances are striking: the mucosa is red, sometimes ulcerated, and bleeds when touched.

The onset of cystitis may be sudden, with suprapubic pain, frequency and scalding on micturition. The patient may sit for hours on the toilet with a constant urge to urinate, passing only an occasional drop of blood-stained urine. If the infection spreads up the ureters to the kidneys there will be pain in the loin with fever and shivering (see p. 59).

There are few physical signs other than tenderness in the suprapubic region.

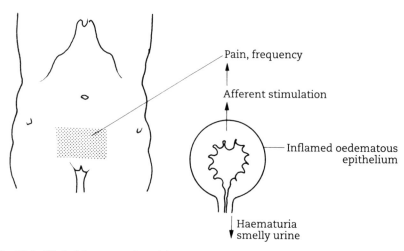

Fig. 15.1 Clinical features of cystitis.

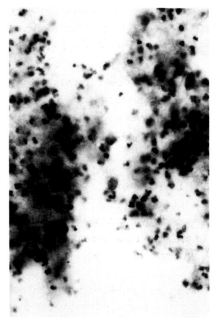

Fig. 15.2 Pus in the urine. Courtesy of Dr Jo Martin.

INVESTIGATIONS

Inspection of the urine shows it to be cloudy: crystal clear urine is never infected. It often smells fishy. Microscopy shows it to be full of pus cells (more than 5 per high power field) and the bacteria can be seen jiggling along the edge of the leucocytes (Fig. 15.2).

The urine is cultured at once using a dip-slide, or cooled and sent as soon as possible to the laboratory where a colony count is performed and antibiotic sensitivities are determined (see p. 13).

TREATMENT

At first one can only guess which organism is responsible for the infection, but a patient who has suffered previous attacks will know which antimicrobial agent made her better last time, and it is sensible to use it again, pending sensitivity studies from the laboratory. Choose a safe and cheap antimicrobial, e.g. trimethoprim, nalidixic acid or nitrofurantoin. Reserve expensive, wide-spectrum antibiotics for severe cases, and use them under microbiological control. If given at the beginning of an attack of cystitis a short course of 1–2 days works as well as a long one: it seldom takes more than 24 h for the antimicrobial to kill the organisms, and perhaps another 24 h for the inflammation to subside.

Making the urine alkaline by giving up to 6 g sodium bicarbonate per day, or a similar amount of potassium citrate, and keeping the urine dilute by drinking 3 litres of fluid a day, makes urination less painful.

FOLLOW-UP

In females it is sometimes difficult to know how diligently to follow up the first attack of acute cystitis. In adult women acute cystitis is so common that a single attack can safely be treated on the lines suggested above. In little girls, and at any age when there have been several attacks, they should be investigated further.

A plain kidney, ureter and bladder (KUB) film to rule out a stone, and an ultrasound scan of the kidneys and bladder are the usual tests: in children a micturating cystogram or ultrasound scan using fizzy water is done to rule out reflux.

Whenever there has been haematuria the urine is examined for malignant cells, and when the acute attack has settled down, a flexible cystoscopy must be performed to rule out a bladder cancer (see p. 166).

If the urine shows pus, but no organisms can be grown in the dip-slide or the laboratory, then one must rule out the other more serious causes of sterile pyuria, namely tuberculosis (see p. 68) and cancer (see p. 161).

CHRONIC CYSTITIS

Repeated attacks of acute cystitis often occur from the same intestinal organism, but if the intestinal flora has been changed as a result of a long course of a broad-spectrum antibiotic, the invading organisms may be resistant to first-line antibiotics, especially if the patient has been sitting around in a hospital bed. Occasionally persistent urinary or vaginal infection seems to become resistant to every type of medication and will only stop when all antibiotics are withheld and the normal vaginal ecology is allowed to restore itself. In this context much has been made of lactobacilli, which vanish from the normal vagina after prolonged treatment with antibiotics, giving rise to the facile suggestion that putting yoghurt into the vagina might prevent urinary infection. Yoghurt contains an entirely different lactobacillus, and does no good at all.

NATURAL DEFENCES OF THE BLADDER

Like a dustbin, the bladder only stays clean if it is emptied regularly (Fig. 15.3). Even when the last drop of urine has been expelled, some bacteria will cling to the urothelial cells after the bladder has been emptied, but these are easily dealt with by the natural bactericidal action of the urothelial cells, a function which is impaired in diabetes and in cancer cells.

Deliberate infection of the bladder with an inoculum of microbes does not cause an infection if the bladder is emptied regularly. However, if the bladder does not empty out completely, because of outflow obstruction or a diverticulum, then a tiny inoculum will divide at body temperature to become millions (see p. 60).

PATHOLOGY OF CHRONIC CYSTITIS

Follicular cystitis. Here repeated infections give rise to collections of lymphocytes under the urothelium which can be recognized as little pale specks on cystoscopy (Fig. 15.4).

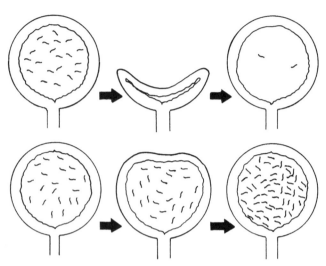

Fig. 15.3 The chief defence of the bladder against infection is to keep itself regularly emptied out completely.

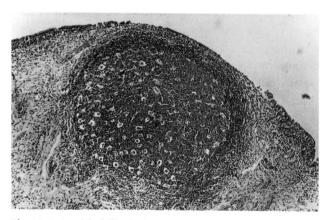

Fig. 15.4 Cystitis follicularis.

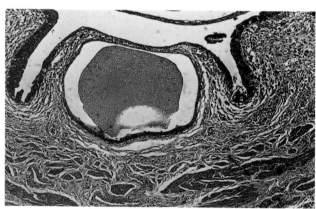

Fig. 15.5 Cystitis cystica.

Cystitis cystica. In severe infections parts of the urothelium are shed, leaving islands of cells which get buried under the regenerating urothelium: these form little cysts under the mucosa which look like little bubbles on cystoscopy — cystitis cystica. This is usually harmless, but if the infection persists, the buried cysts of urothelium undergo metaplasia, secrete mucus, and turn into intestinal mucosa— adenomatous metaplasia—which is the precursor of adenocarcinoma (Fig. 15.5).

MALACOPLAKIA

A variation on this theme is malacoplakia, which forms collections of soft brown lumps in the urothelium which are easily mistaken for cancer (see p. 69).

SQUAMOUS METAPLASIA

Persistent infection, especially when associated with a stone, stricture or schisto-somiasis, causes the urothelium to undergo squamous metaplasia. This is very sinister because it so often progresses to squamous cell cancer (see p. 162).

ALKALINE ENCRUSTED CYSTITIS

Infection with *Proteus mirabilis* can lead to a peculiarly disabling condition in which chronic inflammation accompanied by calcification involves the entire wall of the bladder, converting it into a rigid sphere. Cystoscopy shows stony encrustation all over the wall of the bladder. The urine reeks of ammonia.

HUNNER'S ULCER – INTERSTITIAL CYSTITIS

The cause of this strange condition is still unknown. Clinically, the patient, usually a middle-aged woman, has intense pain whenever the bladder is half-filled. The pain is often felt in one place. There is severe frequency. Cystoscopy at first shows no abnormality, but after the bladder has been filled, and the water is allowed to run out, the urothelium seems to be cracked, and blood trickles out — cascade haemorrhage.

Biopsy shows chronic inflammation of the urothelium and the underlying submucosa. It has been suggested (but not proved) that excess of mast cells are present which secrete histamine. Every year there is a new remedy for this condition but a consistently reliable treatment remains elusive. Some patients are improved if the bladder is stretched; others are better if the 'ulcer' is diathermized; others improve if dimethylsulphoxide (DMSO) is instilled. The condition usually comes back, and the only remedy may be to remove the entire bladder, replacing it with some form of cystoplasty (see p. 172).

INVESTIGATIONS

Every patient with chronic cystitis is investigated by repeated urine cultures, including those for *Mycobacterium tuberculosis* (see p. 66), by intravenous urogram (IVU) and cystoscopy to rule out some mechanical cause for persistent infection. In patients who have travelled in Africa the urine will be examined for the ova of *Schistosoma* (see p. 13). Any cause of stagnation in the urinary tract such as a diverticulum, and any local cause for persistent infection such as a stone or necrosis in a tumour is carefully ruled out.

TREATMENT

Having excluded remediable causes such as a pocket of undrained urine, a stone, tuberculosis or cancer, then we are left with a large number of patients, usually women, with persistent urinary infection. What can be done for them?

A high fluid throughput often helps dramatically, e.g. 3–4 litres/day. This must be combined with frequent emptying of the bladder at least every 2h. Busy women should keep a jug of water on their desk and urinate every 2h by the clock whether they want to go or not.

This simple, if boring, advice will reduce the number of attacks. But when resistance is low, there will be reinfection. Patients who have had many attacks always know when another is coming on, and they also know which medication is likely to cure them. There is no need to withhold treatment until the laboratory has confirmed what the patient already knows: it is far more sensible to supply your patient with a simple antimicrobial, e.g. trimethoprim or nitrofurantoin, to take whenever an attack threatens. This will often nip the episode in the bud, and she will be cured within 24h: if so there is no need to continue medication any longer.

When this simple system does not work a patient may be given long-term methenamine mandelate or hippurate to reinforce their natural defences.

SCHISTOSOMIASIS (BILHARZIASIS)

The trematode flukes *Schistosoma haematobium*, *S. mansoni* and *S. japonicum* are flatworms with a life cycle that involves one stage in a mollusc and another in a vertebrate. The adult flukes are about 5mm in length and live inside human veins, attached to the endothelium by a sucker (Fig. 15.6). The male enfolds the female in a long slit down his belly, hence the name *schisto* (split) and *soma* (body). They were discovered in the portal vein of children by the German pathologist Theodor Bilharz when he was working in Cairo, hence the alternative name bilharziasis. The females lay eggs with terminal spines which vary according to the species (Fig. 15.7).

When the adult flukes are living in the submucosal veins of the bladder their eggs not only bore their way through the urothelium to cause haematuria, but they cause ulceration and polyp formation. The dead eggs calcify, and can be seen on cystoscopy to glisten like grains of sand under the urothelium. The urothelium undergoes squamous metaplasia and eventually may form squamous cell cancer.

A plain X-ray shows the outline of the bladder, lower ureters and vasa deferentia, traced by the millions of dead calcified ova (Fig. 15.8). Low power microscopy of the urine shows the ova (see p. 13).

If the patient urinates into a slow-moving river or irrigation channel, the eggs hatch into *miracidia* which are attracted to fresh-water snails, which they invade. They divide inside the body of the snail, form sporocysts which burst to liberate thousands of minute flukes — *cercariae*. These penetrate the skin of any unwary

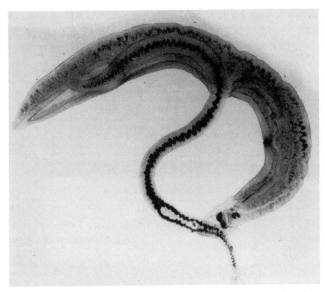

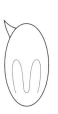 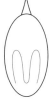 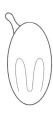

S. mansoni   *S. haematobium*   *S. japonicum*

Fig. 15.6 *Schistosoma haematobium*: pair of adult worms removed from a vein Schistosomes: about 1 cm long.

Fig. 15.7 Bilharzia ova.

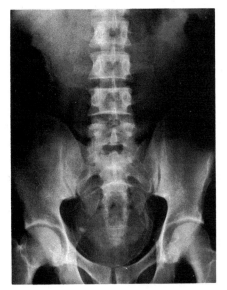

Fig. 15.8 Plain X-ray in schistosomiasis showing calcification in the bladder.

human whose hand or foot happens to be in the water at the right time. It only takes a few seconds for them to enter the skin (Fig. 15.9).

Under the skin, the cercariae cause an itching rash — swimmer's itch. Later they reach the circulation through the lymphatics, and cause a systemic illness — Katagama fever. Finally, adult flukes settle in little veins, which may be anywhere in the body including the brain and spinal cord. In small children large masses congregate and obstruct the portal vein. Schistosomiasis is second only to malaria as a cause of disease, and its eradication depends on the provision of clean water and effective disposal of sewage.

TREATMENT

It is futile to treat infestation if the patient at once returns to work in an infected paddy-field. Treatment consists of a single dose of praziquantel which may be repeated after 1 month. Surgical resection of polypi and ulcers may be necessary, and the squamous cell cancer may require cystectomy (see. p. 171). Obstruction, dilatation and stone formation in the ureters may require appropriate surgery.

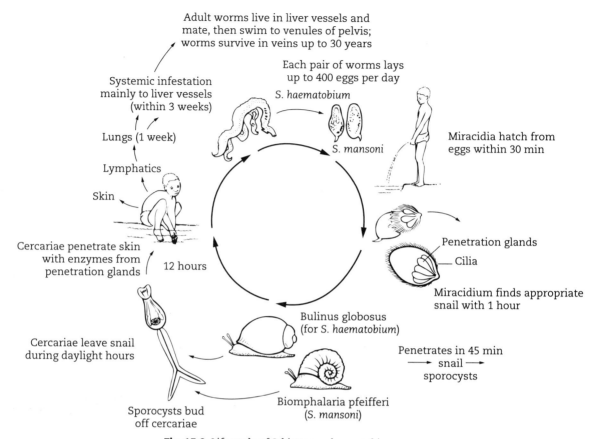

Fig. 15.9 Life cycle of *Schistosoma haematobium*.

STONES IN THE BLADDER

See p. 88.

FURTHER READING

Christmas TJ, Holmes SAV, Hendry WF (1996) Bladder replacement by ileocystoplasty: the final treatment for interstitial cystitis. *Br J Urol* **78**: 69.

Ghoneim MA (1984) Bilharziasis: the lower genitourinary tract. In: Husain I (ed.) *Tropical Urology and Renal Disease*. London, Churchill Livingstone, pp. 261–80.

Hunner GL (1915) A rare type of bladder ulcer in women. *Trans South Surg Gynecol Assoc* **27**: 247.

Redondo-Lopez V, Cook RL, Sobel JD (1990) Emerging role of lactobacilli in the control and maintenance of the vaginal bacterial microflora. *Rev Infect Dis* **12**: 856.

Reid G, Bruce AW (1993) Factors influencing the adhesion of uropathogens to the uroepithelium. *Curr Op Urol* **3**: 21.

Schaeffer AJ (1990) Modifiers of susceptibility to urinary tract infection. *J Urol* **143**: 138.

Thompson AC, Christmas TJ (1996) Interstitial cystitis—an update. *Br J Urol* **78**: 813.

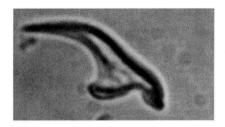

Bladder Cancer

Because the bladder is lined by urothelium its neoplasms are nearly always transitional cell carcinomas, but if urothelium undergoes metaplasia into squamous or glandular epithelium (as happens with prolonged irritation or infection) then squamous cell cancer and adenocarcinoma can occur. Secondary cancer is sometimes seen from direct invasion from a primary tumour in the colon, rectum or uterus.

CANCER OF THE UROTHELIUM

AETIOLOGY

In 1894 Rehn noticed that workers in the aniline dye industry were developing an unduly large number of cancers of the bladder. Hueper subsequently showed that the cause was neither aniline, nor the finished dyestuffs, but a group of intermediate nitrophenols (Fig. 16.1) of which the most dangerous were β-naphthylamine and benzidine. These substances were also present in tobacco smoke and other industries including rubber moulding and the coal–gas industry. All these industries have now eliminated these chemicals from their factories, but tobacco

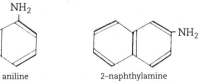

aniline   2–naphthylamine   4,4–diaminodiphenyl (benzidine)

Fig. 16.1 Aniline and its carcinogenic relatives.

161

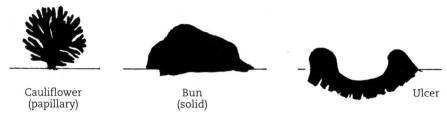

Cauliflower
(papillary)

Bun
(solid)

Ulcer

Fig. 16.2 Macroscopic features of bladder cancer.

smoking continues to be a major hazard. In other parts of the world the prolonged irritation of the urothelium by schistosomiasis continues to be a major cause, perhaps added to by tobacco smoking (see p. 158).

PATHOLOGY

Bladder tumours may be single or multiple, and like all cancers, can take the shape of a cauliflower, an ulcer or a solid lump (Fig. 16.2). Truly benign papillomas are exceedingly rare, and it is a pity that the term is often misused for the papillary forms of cancer. There are three grades of malignancy, G1, G2 and G3; G3 being the worst (Fig. 16.3).

SQUAMOUS CARCINOMA

Squamous changes are often seen in patches in G3 transitional cell cancers, and carry a bad prognosis. Pure squamous cancers have a thick layer of white keratin over them.

ADENOCARCINOMA

The glandular metaplasia seen in chronic infection (see p. 156) and exstrophy (see p. 149) may proceed to adenocarcinoma. Adenocarcinoma also arises in the vestige of the fetal allantois, the urachus, as a cherry-like lump at the top of the bladder.

SPREAD OF BLADDER CANCER

Direct spread
Cancer may invade the surrounding fat and adjacent organs but never seems to cross Denonvilliers' fascia into the rectum, although cancer of the rectum appears to have no difficulty crossing into the bladder.

Implantation
Bladder cancer may be seeded into the urethra and possibly onto the opposite wall of the bladder—kiss cancer.

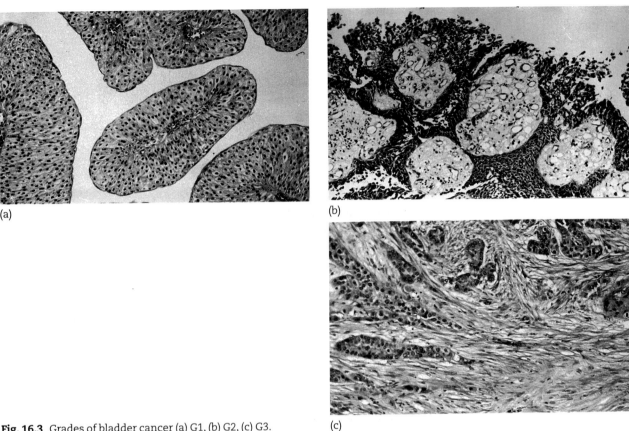

(a)

(b)

(c)

Fig. 16.3 Grades of bladder cancer (a) G1, (b) G2, (c) G3.

Lymphatic spread

Once a bladder cancer has invaded the detrusor muscle it finds a rich plexus of lymphatics, and quickly spreads into the nodes along the internal iliac artery and up along the aorta. There is also a direct connection between these lymphatics and the bone marrow of the pelvis, the upper end of the femur, and the lower vertebrae.

Systemic spread

Metastases are occasionally seen in the lungs, liver or brain, but they are rare when compared with other cancers of the viscera.

STAGING OF BLADDER CANCER

The International Union against Cancer (UICC) uses the TNM system of staging, which is intended to enable different centres to compare their results (Fig. 16.4).

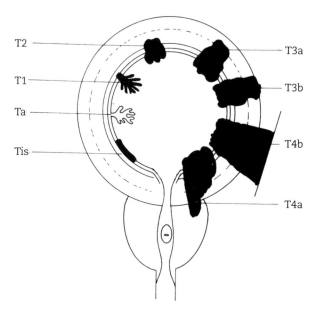

Fig. 16.4 Staging of bladder cancer.

T staging system takes into account the evidence on which the depth of invasion has been assessed; e.g. the prefix T means a clinical guess, based on the assessment at the time of cystoscopy. A lower case p is added when there is a deep biopsy showing enough muscle to tell whether it has been invaded or not. An upper case P means that part or all of the bladder muscle has been removed.

N staging—the assessment of lymph node involvement (N)—is always guesswork unless the lymph nodes have been removed surgically and sent for histological examination. Computed tomography (CT) and magnetic resonance imaging (MRI) can detect the larger metastases with much less accuracy.

M staging—the detection of visceral metastases—depends on chest X-rays and ultrasound scanning of the liver.

The differences in the methods used to stage bladder cancer make it necessary to be wary of comparing the results of treatment by total cystectomy (where there is pathological evidence of depth of invasion and lymph node involvement) with those of radiotherapy, or chemotherapy, which can only be based on biopsies, with CT and ultrasound scanning, and tend to underestimate the stage.

CLINICAL FEATURES

SCREENING OF SYMPTOMLESS PATIENTS
Patients thought to be at risk, e.g. in the chemical and rubber industry, have their

urine screened for malignant cells (see p. 12). The cytological diagnosis of cancer depends on recognizing large, multinucleated malignant cells in the urine (Fig. 16.5). If the tumour is G1 (well differentiated), the cells may go unrecognized unless by chance a broken-off frond of a papillary tumour is discovered. Automated flow cytometry measures the nuclear:cytoplasm ratio in large numbers of cells, thus avoiding observer error.

Symptoms

More than 80% of patients with bladder cancer present with haematuria (Fig. 16.6), which is the reason why every patient with haematuria must be cystoscoped. This rule applies whether the blood has been seen with the naked eye, or found by the stix test (see p. 10). The problem is that the other 20% have not noticed blood in their urine and it is important to be aware of the other symptoms that should raise suspicion.

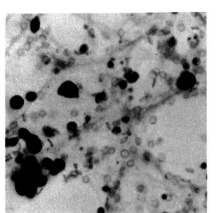

Fig. 16.5 Malignant cells in the urine.

'Cystitis' with sterile pyuria. The urothelium around a bladder tumour is often inflamed, and the patient may then have frequency and pain on voiding, just like ordinary cystitis. The clue is to find many 'pus cells' in the urine on microscopy, but no microorganisms in culture. Pus cells can look very like leucocytes on ordinary microscopy. Sterile pyuria equals cancer until proven otherwise.

The decoy prostate. Most bladder cancers occur in elderly men, in whom irritability of the bladder often suggests prostatic outflow obstruction (see p. 197). To avoid this pitfall every man with 'prostatism' must have his urine tested for blood and cytology, and before prostatectomy the bladder must always be carefully examined to rule out a small cancer.

Anaemia. Continued loss of blood in the urine sometimes brings a patient to the doctor with anaemia, out of all proportion to the size of the cancer.

Urinary infection. Infection occurring for no obvious reason in an elderly patient, particularly a heavy smoker, should be regarded with suspicion: it may be arising in the necrotic superficial part of a solid tumour (see p. 157).

Pain. This usually means that the cancer has invaded outside the bladder.

Physical signs

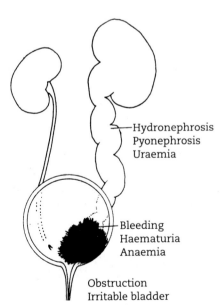

Hydronephrosis
Pyonephrosis
Uraemia

Bleeding
Haematuria
Anaemia

Obstruction
Irritable bladder

Fig. 16.6 Clinical features of bladder cancer.

There are usually none, except in the rare tumour that arises from the urachus, when a hard mass is felt between the symphysis and the umbilicus. Otherwise if a mass can be felt, it signifies gross extension of the cancer.

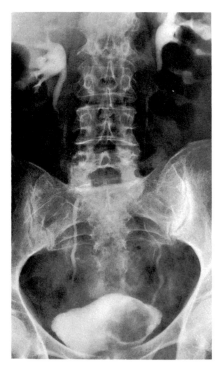

Fig. 16.7 IVU in bladder cancer showing large filling defect.

Investigations

Doctors should respond to the finding of haematuria almost with a knee-jerk: haematuria = intravenous urogram (IVU) + cystoscopy. The IVU often shows a filling defect in the bladder (Fig. 16.7), and if a ureter is obstructed, it usually means the muscle near the ureteric orifice is invaded by tumour, and hence the growth is T2 or worse.

Ultrasound scanning of the bladder may also show a large tumour (Fig. 16.8) and an even better picture is obtained with an ultrasound probe passed per urethram. But neither of these tests replaces cystoscopy.

Cystoscopy is the essential investigation. A flexible cystoscopy is quick and painless and does not require admission to hospital. If a tumour has already been detected in the IVU the flexible cystoscopy can be bypassed and arrangements made for cystoscopy under anaesthesia.

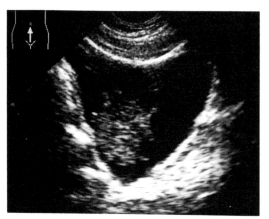

Fig. 16.8 Ultrasound image showing bladder tumour. Courtesy of Dr W. Hately.

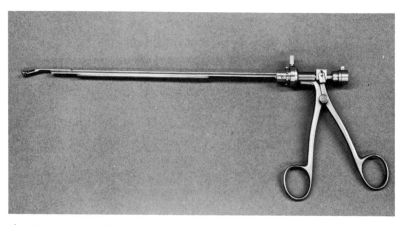

Fig. 16.9 Storz cup biopsy forceps.

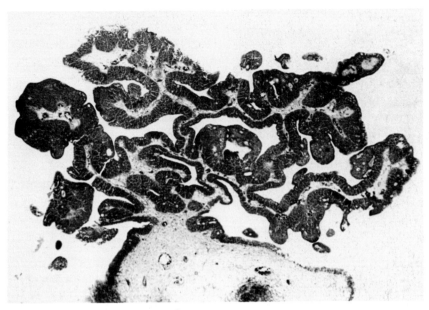

Fig. 16.10 Biopsy taken with cup forceps.

CYSTOSCOPY AND BIOPSY

A biopsy is obtained with the resectoscope or a cup forceps (Fig. 16.9). It must include muscle from the base of the tumour to establish its depth of invasion (Fig. 16.10). Bimanual palpation is performed to assess induration after the removal of the tumour which might indicate deep muscle invasion, e.g. T3.

TREATMENT OF BLADDER CANCER

Carcinoma in situ (G3 pTis)

This usually presents as 'cystitis' in a heavy smoker, who has seldom noticed haematuria. 'Pus cells' are present in the urine, which is sterile on culture (Fig. 16.11). Malignant cells are present in the cytological examination. On cystoscopy the bladder may perhaps look a little inflamed. Biopsies of the urothelium confirm the diagnosis. The condition often responds completely to instillations of bacille Calmette–Guérin (BCG) (see p. 169) but must be kept under close review because it very easily turns into G3 invasive cancer.

Ta and T1 urothelial cancer

These tumours are initially removed by the resectoscope (Fig. 16.12), or, having

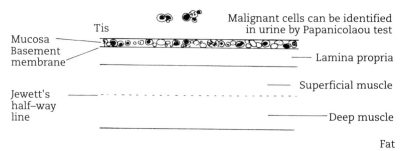

Fig. 16.11 Flat carcinoma *in situ*.

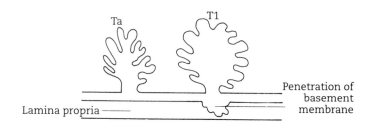

Fig. 16.12 Ta and T1 carcinoma of the bladder.

Fig. 16.13 Small papillary tumour removed with resectoscope loop.

removed two or three with an adequate base of muscle (Fig. 16.13), the remainder are coagulated with the diathermy ball (Fig. 16.14). The same coagulation can be obtained using the neodymium–yttrium/aluminium/garnet (YAG) laser (Fig. 16.15). Patients are all carefully followed up at regular intervals by cytology and flexible cystoscopy. Recurrences are treated by transurethral resection or coagulation.

TRANSURETHRAL RESECTION OF A BLADDER TUMOUR

If the IVU or flexible cystoscopy has revealed a bulky tumour, serum should be sent for grouping in case blood is needed. The operation requires general or spinal anaesthetic, and can be prolonged and often quite difficult. The object is to cut away the 'bush' to reveal the 'stalk' of the cancer (Fig. 16.16). This is thoroughly coagulated to control bleeding, and removed down to the deeper layers of the detrusor muscle. The 'bush' and the 'stalk' are sent separately to the laboratory so that the pathologist can tell how deeply the muscle is invaded. After all the bleeding has been stopped, a catheter is left in for a day or two. Possible complications include perforation of the wall of the bladder, absorption of irrigating fluid, and bleeding (see transurethral resection of the prostate, p. 199).

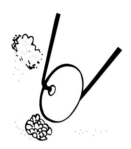

Fig. 16.14 Small papillary tumour coagulated with roly-ball electrode.

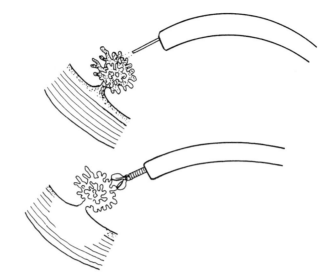

Fig. 16.15 Small papillary tumour coagulated with YAG laser through flexible cystoscope.

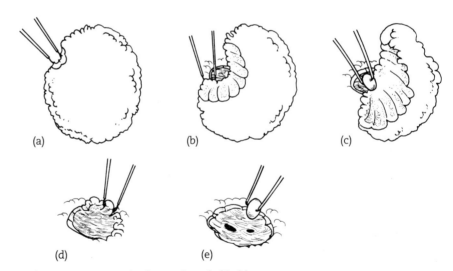

(a)

(b)

(c)

(d)

(e)

Fig. 16.16 Transurethral resection of a bladder tumour.

ADJUVANT TREATMENT

When there are very frequent and multiple recurrences the patient is given a course of intravesical instillations of BCG or some other antimitotic agent such as mitomycin, adriamycin or epodyl. The most useful of these is BCG, but it causes a more or less painful cystitis. The response to the first course of BCG may be permanent but usually repeated courses are required. Occasionally the mild form of tuberculosis which is caused by the attenuated BCG leads to hepatitis, and may call for antituberculous therapy (see p. 69).

Mitomycin treatment may cause an allergic reaction if it gets into contact with skin.

G3 SUPERFICIAL CANCERS

The exception to this rather conservative policy is the uncommon G3 superficial papillary tumour which carries such a bad prognosis that it is generally treated as if it were already invading the wall of the bladder (see below).

T2, T3 invasive cancer

Most of these invasive cancers are G3. The distinction between T2 and T3 is somewhat artificial, being based on an imaginary half-way line in the bladder muscle (Figs 16.17, 16.18). Although the T2 cancers have a slightly better prognosis than T3 the difference is slight when compared with the dramatic worsening in survival once muscle begins to be invaded.

There are three main methods of treatment but there is no agreement as to how best to combine them.

TOTAL CYSTECTOMY

The operation (see p. 171) has the advantage of giving a true P staging, and can be combined with removal of pelvic lymph nodes which may not only provide an accurate N staging, but may be curative. A new bladder can be made for the patient out of small or large bowel, and it is sometimes possible to protect the nerve supply to the penis and preserve potency.

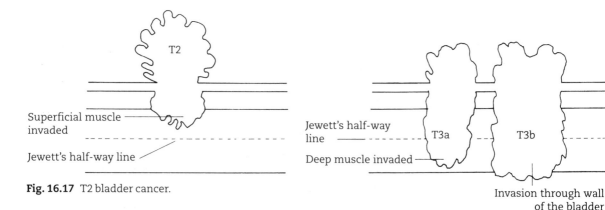

Fig. 16.17 T2 bladder cancer.

Fig. 16.18 T3 bladder cancers.

RADIOTHERAPY

About half of the G3 muscle-invading cancers will disappear completely after a course of 5500 cGy from the linear accelerator. There is at present no way of predicting which cancer will respond, although the presence of squamous metaplasia and staining for β-human chorionic gonadotrophin in the tissue strongly suggest that it will not. In the UK and Canada it is usual to try radiotherapy first, and to perform 'salvage' cystectomy only when the cancer fails to go away completely or comes back later. Elsewhere early radical cystectomy is preferred. The disadvantage of radiotherapy is that if cystectomy is needed later on, because of persistent or recurrent cancer, then it is more difficult to construct a new bladder, and the patient usually requires an ileal loop diversion (see p. 172). The disadvantage of performing cystectomy as the method of first choice is that it denies the patient the possible adjuvant effect of radiation, and the chance of escaping cystectomy altogether.

COMBINATION CHEMOTHERAPY

Various combinations of chemotherapeutic agents have been used which may give 'complete remission' in about half of the cases, but the treatment is very toxic and the response seldom prolonged. In most centres these regimes are reserved for patients who refuse or are not fit to undergo cystectomy, or as part of a combination with radiotherapy and 'salvage' cystectomy.

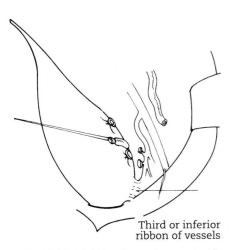

Third or inferior ribbon of vessels

Fig. 16.19 Dividing the main vessels of the bladder.

TOTAL CYSTECTOMY

This is still a very major operation, and the patient needs to understand fully its grave implications. Nearly every male is rendered impotent, and it is essential to discuss all the implications and problems that are associated with various forms of urinary diversion (see p. 172).

PREPARATION

The bowel is prepared with a high fluid intake and antibiotics. Anaemia is corrected by appropriate transfusion. Smoking is forbidden to minimize chest infection. Six units of blood are cross-matched. The site for the ileal conduit is carefully selected and marked, using a dummy bag containing water.

STEPS OF THE OPERATION

All the lymph nodes are dissected off the aorta, common and internal iliac vessels on each side and sent for frozen section, for if they are involved, the operation may more appropriately be abandoned. All the vessels supplying the bladder from the internal iliac artery are divided between ligatures, one after the other (Fig. 16.19). The ureters are divided about 5 cm away from the bladder (Fig. 16.20).

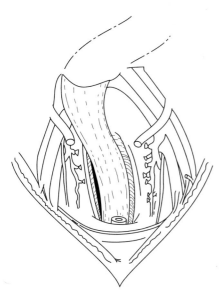

Fig. 16.20 The empty pelvis after the bladder has been removed.

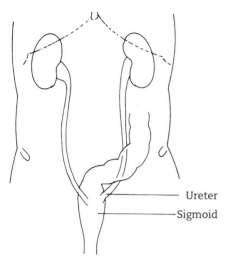

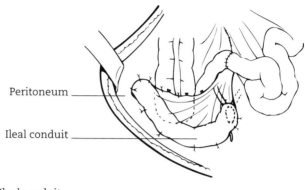

Fig. 16.22 Ileal conduit.

Fig. 16.21 Ureterosigmoidostomy.

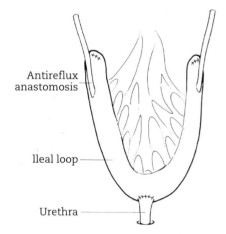

Fig. 16.23 Neocystoplasty by Camey's method.

When there are multiple tumours, with the chance of recurrent cancer in the urethra, the urethra is removed *en bloc* with the bladder and prostate.

Urinary diversion

URETEROSIGMOIDOSTOMY

This is the oldest technique: the ureters are led through tunnels in the wall of the sigmoid to prevent faeces from refluxing up them to the kidney (Fig. 16.21). Unfortunately this operation was frequently followed by infection, and absorption of urine from the colon led to hyperchloraemic acidosis and renal failure. It has been almost entirely abandoned.

ILEAL CONDUIT

The ureters are anastomosed to one end of an isolated loop of ileum whose other end is led onto the skin to form a urostomy which is fitted with an adhesive bag (Fig. 16.22). Care must be taken in choosing the site for the stoma: it must not rub against the belt or lie in a scar or crease or else the bag will come unstuck.

NEOCYSTOPLASTY

After removing the bladder, a new one is constructed out of intestine. Numerous different methods are in use, but they all share certain principles. Initially, the bowel is open and closed in such a way that powerful peristaltic waves cannot generate an increase in pressure, and as a rule precautions are taken to prevent reflux of urine from the new bladder up the ureters (Fig. 16.23).

If the urethra has been removed, a stoma is made onto the skin which is designed to be continent, so that the patient empties it from time to time with a catheter (Fig. 16.24).

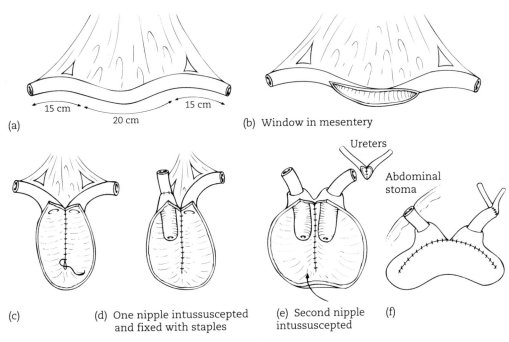

(a)

(b) Window in mesentery

Ureters

Abdominal stoma

(c)

(d) One nipple intussuscepted and fixed with staples

(e) Second nipple intussuscepted

(f)

Fig. 16.24 Kock's continent pouch.

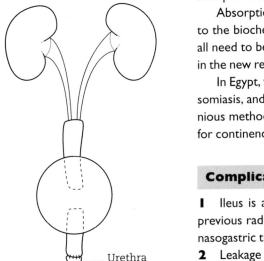

Fig. 16.25 A Kock pouch may be anastomosed to the urethra.

If the urethra has not been removed, the reservoir can be sewn onto the stump of urethra and in many cases normal voiding is established (Fig. 16.25).

Absorption of urine from the bowel used to make the new bladder still leads to the biochemical complication of hyperchloraemic acidosis, and these patients all need to be carefully followed to make sure that infection and stone formation in the new reservoir is detected and treated.

In Egypt, where cystectomy is required for squamous cell cancer after schistosomiasis, and the poor farm labourers cannot afford adhesive appliances, an ingenious method of diversion has been devised that makes use of the anal sphincter for continence (Fig. 16.26).

Complications of cystectomy

1 Ileus is always prolonged after cystectomy, the more so if there has been previous radiation treatment. During this time the bowel is kept deflated with a nasogastric tube or gastrostomy.

2 Leakage from the anastomoses between the ureters and the new bladder or ileal conduit, or breakdown of the elaborate suture lines of the reconstructed bladder, call for strict vigilance in the early postoperative period, and it is not uncommon to have to revise the reservoir.

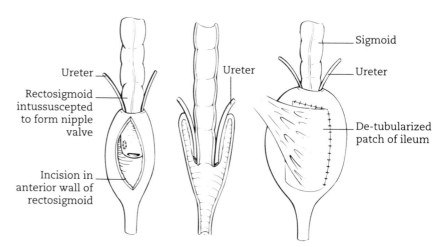

Fig. 16.26 Ghoneim's continent diversion.

3 Pulmonary infection may require physiotherapy and antibiotics.
4 Deep venous thrombosis and pulmonary embolism are common complications and call for the usual prevention.

Carcinoma of the urachus

This is very uncommon, and is almost the only indication for partial cystectomy. The tumour presents as a small cherry-like swelling at the top of the bladder. Outside it is a much larger mass (Fig. 16.27). Biopsy shows adenocarcinoma. It is treated by a wide excision that takes all the triangle of tissue from the umbilicus down to the upper part of the bladder as well as all the regional lymph nodes. The small residual bladder is closed, but enlarges to its former capacity within a few weeks (Fig. 16.28).

PALLIATION

When treatment has failed we are faced with an elderly patient, who has to void blood-stained urine with pain and difficulty every few minutes by day and night. Pain and infection in recurrent necrotic tumour makes the patient even more ill. Cancer of the bladder seldom brings a quick and merciful end from metastases.

Surgeons can do much towards the relief of suffering. A palliative urinary diversion with a ureterosigmoidostomy or an ileal conduit may stop the painful frequency. Palliative radiotherapy may stop bleeding and control pain. Pain-relieving medication should be provided at the control of the patient, i.e. when needed, not according to the hour, for pain knows no clock.

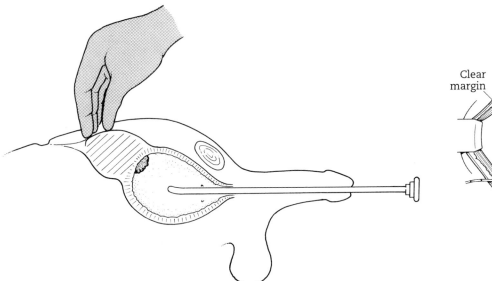

Fig. 16.27 Carcinoma of the urachus.

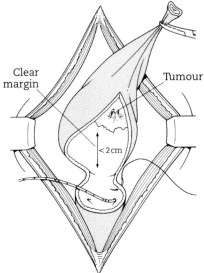

Fig. 16.28 Subtotal cystectomy for carcinoma of the urachus.

In the end you are the doctor. You may be embarrassed and reluctant to visit your patients because you are ashamed of having so little to offer. Do not be mistaken: you can provide something of special value merely by being there from time to time. You can at least show that you are still the patient's friend, and that you care.

FURTHER READING

Chersi D, Stewart LA, Parmar MKB *et al.* (1995) Does neoadjuvant cisplatin-based chemotherapy improve the survival of patients with locally advanced bladder cancer: a meta-analysis of individual patient data from randomized clinical trials. *Br J Urol* **75**: 206.

Chinegwundoh FI, Kaisary AV (1996) Polymorphism and smoking in bladder carcinogenesis. *Br J Urol* **77**: 672–5.

Frazier HA, Robertson JE, Paulson DR (1992) Complications of radical cystectomy and urinary diversion: a retrospective review of 675 cases in two decades. *J Urol* **148**: 1402.

Hueper WC, Wiley FH, Wolfe HD (1938) Experimental production of bladder tumors in dogs by administration of beta-naphthylamine. *J Industr Hyg Toxicol* **20**: 46.

Jenkins BJ, Martin JE, Baithun SI, Zuk RJ, Oliver RTD, Blandy JP (1990) Prediction of response to radiotherapy in invasive bladder cancer. *Br J Urol* **65**: 345.

Jewett HJ, Strong GH (1946) Infiltrating carcinoma of the bladder: relation of depth of penetration of the bladder wall to incidence of local extension and metastases. *J Urol* **55**: 366.

Morales A, Nickel JC, Wilson JWL (1992) Dose–reponse of bacillus Calmette–Guérin in the treatment of superficial bladder cancer. *J Urol* **147**: 1256.

Nouri AME, Darakhshan F, Cannell H, Paris AMI, Oliver RTD (1996) The relevance of p53 mutations in urological malignancies: possible implications for bladder cancer. *Br J Urol* **78**: 337–44 (review).

Rehn L (1895) Blasengeschwultse bei fuchsinarbeitern. *Arch Clin Chir* **50**: 588.

Shirai T, Fradet Y, Huland H *et al.* (1995) The etiology of bladder cancer—are there any new clues or predictors of behaviour? *Int J Urol* **2** (suppl. 2) 64.

Silverman DT, Hartge P, Morrison AS, Devesa SS (1992) Epidemiology of bladder cancer. *Hematol Oncol Clin N Am* **6**: 1.

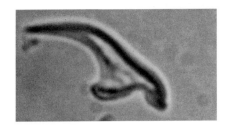

The Bladder: Disorders of Micturition

DIURESIS

POLYDIPSIA

Some patients who are otherwise perfectly normal, form the habit of drinking an excessive amount of fluid: what goes in must come out. The diagnosis is made by asking the patient to keep a diary of their input and output of fluid.

DIABETES MELLITUS

Nothing is more simple than to test for glucose in the urine.

DIABETES INSIPIDUS

The anterior pituitary may fail to secrete antidiuretic hormone so that the patient is unable to concentrate urine. In children the enormous output of urine may lead to dilatation of the entire urinary tract.

RENAL TUBULAR DISORDERS

The renal tubules fail to concentrate urine for three main reasons:

1 Obstruction. In bilateral hydronephrosis there is loss of the renal papillae so that water and salt are not reabsorbed. The urine is pale and of fixed specific gravity: the patient may be dehydrated and short of salt.

2 Old age. The pituitary fails to secrete the usual amount of antidiuretic hormone at night. At the same time the inferior vena cava fails to contract when the patient lies down, and there is continued secretion of the atrial natriuretic hormone. There is in addition very often a mild degree of heart failure and the fluid retained in the day as oedema in the lower limbs, is excreted at night. The diagnosis is easily made by asking the patient to keep a diary of the volumes of

urine he or she passes at night. A small dose of desmopressin, e.g. 10–20 μg at bedtime, may give the patient a good night's rest.

3 Sickle cell disease. Both homozygous and heterozygous forms of the disease may give rise to loss of function of the renal papillae (see p. 52). Patients are found to have urine of a fixed specific gravity and often a mild diuresis.

NEUROPATHY

OVERSTIMULATION OF THE AFFERENT ARM OF THE MICTURITION REFLEX

Anything which makes the lining of the bladder more sensitive may provoke detrusor contraction before the bladder is full (Fig. 17.1), e.g. a stone, infection or carcinoma. At its worst there may be a contraction of the detrusor which the patient cannot inhibit, causing one form of urge incontinence. Urodynamic studies (see p. 142) will show uninhibited detrusor contractions, a normal flow rate, normal sphincters but a small voided volume.

EXCESSIVE CENTRAL FACILITATION

Everyone who has faced an important examination will know that anxiety can cause frequency (Fig. 17.2). In major anxiety states frequency and even urge incontinence are common, and can make life intolerable. As a general rule this type of frequency only occurs in the daytime, in contrast to the frequency caused by irritation of the urothelium (above).

LACK OF CENTRAL INHIBITION OF THE REFLEX (Fig. 17.3)

Bed-wetting

Babies, like puppies and kittens, have to learn to inhibit the reflex emptying of the

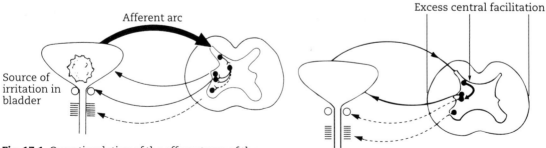

Fig. 17.1 Overstimulation of the afferent arm of the micturition reflex.

Fig. 17.2 Excessive central facilitation.

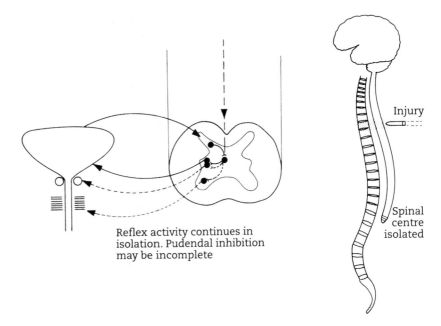

Reflex activity continues in
isolation. Pudendal inhibition
may be incomplete

Injury

Spinal
centre
isolated

Fig. 17.3 Lack of central inhibition.

full bladder until time and place are convenient. In some children this learning process is delayed: many children who wet the bed seem to sleep unusually deeply. In practice the difficulty is to know how far to take investigations of an otherwise normal child, since bed-wetting is quite normal up to the age of 5 or 6; however, the urine should always be tested to exclude infection. Treatment exploits four principles: a small dose of pituitary antidiuretic hormone is given (desmopressin 5–20 µg at bedtime). Imipramine in appropriate doses may work by lightening sleep, or by soothing the detrusor. A buzzer which sounds when soaked with urine may establish a conditioned reflex provided the child is woken up and taken to the lavatory. Fortunately most children grow out of bed-wetting.

Senility

One humiliating feature of old age is incontinence of urine. A brief visit to a residential home for older people is enough to show that we are ineffective in dealing with it. There is usually a mixture of causes:
1   Lack of central inhibition, e.g. after a stroke.
2   Unawareness of a full bladder.
3   Detrusor instability (see p. 180).
4   Immobility, from arthritis or weakness, preventing the person from getting to the lavatory on time.

The management is difficult and takes patience. A friendly reminder at regular intervals may encourage emptying of the bladder before there is an accident.

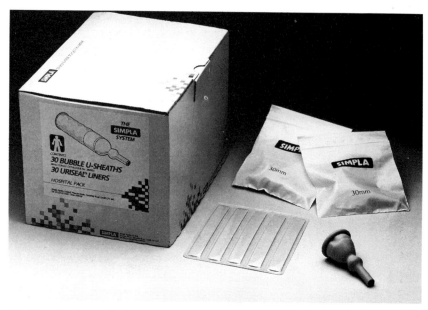

Fig. 17.4 Condom urinal.

Underpants with an absorbent pad placed outside a layer of unwettable material may keep the skin relatively dry, but the pads must be changed regularly, or they stink of ammonia. For men there are various urinals which fit the penis to collect the urine (Fig. 17.4). An indwelling catheter may be the last resort.

HIGH SPINAL CORD LESIONS

Messages from higher centres may be prevented from descending to S2, S3. As a result there may be no coordination between detrusor contraction and relaxation of the sphincters (see p. 141). The detrusor contracts but the sphincters stay shut. The detrusor contracts more powerfully and the intravesical pressure rises, causing dilatation of the ureters and obstructive uropathy (see p. 62) (Fig. 17.5). There is a critical intravesical voiding pressure above which upper tract damage occurs, and it is remarkably low, e.g. about $40\,cmH_2O$.

Trauma

When the spinal cord lesion is caused by trauma, e.g. a gun-shot wound, there is a period of spinal shock during which oedema makes the lesion seem worse than it really is. Hence at first no irreversible steps are taken, and the bladder is merely kept empty by regular intermittent catheterization.

When enough time has elapsed to allow the spinal shock to recover, urodynamic measurements are made. They may show that the sphincters are failing to relax in harmony with the contraction of the detrusor. There are now five possible options:

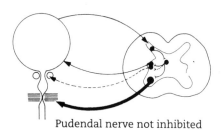

Pudendal nerve not inhibited

Fig. 17.5 Failure of the external sphincter to relax when the detrusor contracts.

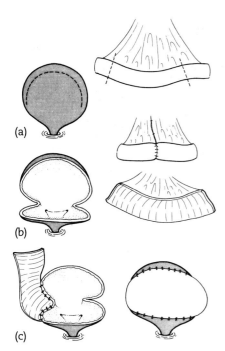

Fig. 17.6 Clam cystoplasty.

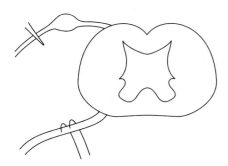

Fig. 17.7 Nerve root division and stimulation.

1 Intermittent self-catheterization. The patient learns to pass a catheter regularly to keep the bladder empty. Unfortunately, with high spinal cord lesions the detrusor may contract spontaneously even when the bladder is almost empty, so that the patient is wet, and a dangerously high pressure may be generated inside the bladder.

2 Sphincterotomy. The three parts of the sphincter in the male may be divided with a resectoscope one at a time, in the hope that the bladder will empty at a less than dangerously high pressure. Sometimes sphincterotomy of the bladder neck is enough to allow the patient to remain dry. More often it is necessary to divide the supramembranous and external sphincters as well.

3 Cystoplasty. When there is a very high pressure inside the bladder, it is opened like a clam, and a length of ileum is isolated, slit open, unfolded, and sewn into the gap (Fig. 17.6). When the detrusor contracts the patch of bowel balloons out and the pressure does not rise. This protects the kidneys and in some cases, with the assistance of a partial sphincterotomy, continence can be preserved. The patient may have to empty the bladder by intermittent clean self-catheterization.

4 Nerve root division and stimulation. The afferent nerve roots to S2, S3 may be divided, and the efferent nerve roots may be fitted with stimulators that enable the bladder to contract at will. These are all very new procedures that are undergoing trial and development (Fig. 17.7).

5 Diversion. Unfortunately many patients, particularly those with weakness of the upper limbs, and those who are confined to a wheelchair, are not able to practice intermittent clean self-catheterization. For them an ileal conduit or a form of continent diversion may be the most appropriate solution (see p. 172).

LESIONS OF THE BLADDER CENTRE AT S2, S3

Destruction of S2, S3

Because the S2, S3 segments are situated in the conus medullaris at the tip of the spinal cord, just opposite the disc between T12 and L1 vertebrae, they are frequently injured in accidents. In practice to show whether they are intact or not there are three useful tests (Fig. 17.8):

1 The bulbospongiosus reflex, i.e. pinch the glans penis and feel for a contraction of the bulbospongiosus muscle (Fig. 17.9).

2 Cystometrogram. The return of detrusor contractions (which can be provoked with ice-cold water) means that the reflex arc must be intact (see p. 142).

3 Electromyography. When the S2, S3 segments are destroyed there are no action potentials in the levator ani (see p. 143).

Management

Without a reflex arc to drive it, the bladder is converted into an inert floppy bag which fills up and then starts to leak—overflow incontinence. It can sometimes be

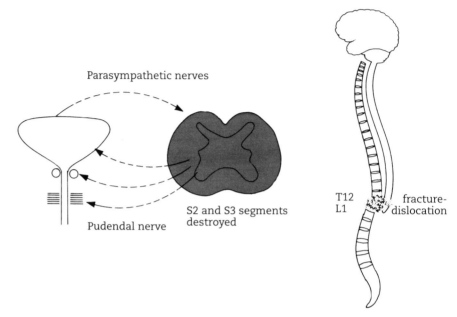

Fig. 17.8 Destruction of the S2, S3 segments, e.g. by fracture.

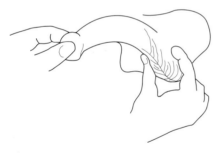

Fig. 17.9 Bulbospongiosus reflex.

emptied by suprapubic compression although this may raise the pressure inside the bladder and threaten the upper tracts. Emptying may be incomplete and infection often develops in the residual urine. For these reasons patients are usually advised to use intermittent clean self-catheterization at least twice a day.

Irritation of S2, S3

Cauda equina lesions

The most medial fibres of the cauda equina going to and from S2, S3 may be irritated by a central prolapse of a lumbar intervertebral disc, causing a characteristic combination of frequency and impotence. Removal of the offending disc may cure both disorders (Fig. 17.10).

Lesions of the pelvic autonomic nerves

Similar clinical conditions may be caused by lesions of the pelvic parasympathetic nerves: they may be torn in fractures of the pelvis or removed in the course of radical surgery for cancer. Their myelin sheaths are frequently involved in diabetes mellitus and the Shy–Drager syndrome. The result is a big floppy bladder with an inert detrusor.

If the presacral sympathetic nerves are affected by these conditions the seminal vesicles and bladder neck do not contract during ejaculation with the

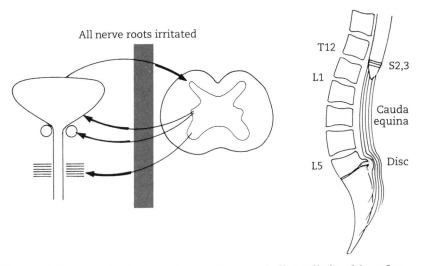

All nerve roots irritated

T12

S2,3

L1

Cauda
equina

L5   Disc

Fig. 17.10 Cauda equina lesion irritating afferent and efferent limbs of the reflex arc.

result that there is retrograde emission of semen, but the detrusor function is unaffected.

DETRUSOR INSTABILITY

By urodynamic convention, when no cause can be found for uninhibited contractions of the detrusor, it is called detrusor instability, so it is a diagnosis that can be made only by exclusion. A degree of detrusor instability is found in many normal people if subjected to careful urodynamic studies. Since these detrusor contractions can sometimes be precipitated by coughing or straining, if they are followed by incontinence the diagnosis can easily be confused with stress incontinence (see below). At present the cause of detrusor instability is not known, with the result that there are many theories and many types of treatment, none of which are very effective.

MECHANICAL LESIONS OF THE BLADDER OUTLET

OBSTRUCTION

Whether the cause is neuropathic failure of the sphincters to relax in harmony with the contraction of the detrusor (see p. 185), obstruction by enlargement of the prostate (see p. 195), or a stricture of the urethra (see p. 232) there are two phases to the response of the detrusor.

Compensatory hypertrophy. The detrusor responds to the demand for a stronger contraction by an increase in the size and strength of its smooth muscle fibres, and a coarsening of the network in which they are arranged — trabeculation (Fig. 17.11). The urothelium begins to bulge out through the gaps in the network forming saccules which eventually balloon right outside the bladder as diverticula.

During this phase of compensatory hypertrophy unstable detrusor contractions occur, generating a high pressure, and sometimes leading to incontinence of urine. This is one form of instability which can be reversed by removing the cause of the obstruction.

Detrusor failure. Like any muscle that has to go on working against abnormal resistance, the detrusor eventually gives up. Instead of emptying the bladder completely, it slowly permits the quantity of residual urine to increase. The time comes when detrusor contractions disappear entirely from the cystometrogram, perhaps because any last weak efforts of the muscle are absorbed by the thin-walled diverticula. The flow is reduced to a trickle, and then only when the pres-

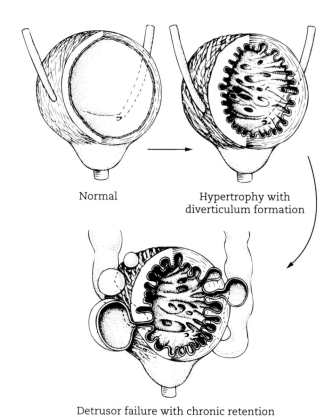

Normal   Hypertrophy with
                          diverticulum formation

Detrusor failure with chronic retention

Fig. 17.11 Compensatory hypertrophy of the detrusor.

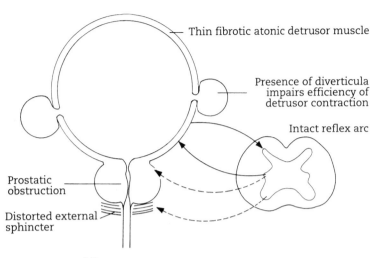

Fig. 17.12 Detrusor failure.

sure in the bladder is increased by abdominal straining or coughing. Before long the huge floppy bladder dribbles without control — retention with overflow (Fig. 17.12).

Such a bladder never recovers its normal function even with prolonged drainage and removal of the obstruction. The residual urine easily becomes infected. Stones or cancer may develop silently in the large diverticula (see p. 20).

DETRUSOR–SPHINCTER DYSSYNERGIA

Detrusor contraction without synchronous relaxation of the sphincters is easily understood when there is an obvious neurological disorder, but it also occurs from time to time in otherwise normal people. Urodynamic studies show a high detrusor pressure, but one or more parts of the sphincter fail to relax. The most common form is seen in middle-aged men, where the α-adrenergic fibres of the bladder neck fail to relax. This can be successfully treated with α-blockers such as prazosin and indoramin. If this gives a good clinical result, the fibres may be divided by transurethral incision of the bladder neck (see p. 199).

When it is the striated muscle component of the sphincter that fails to relax, the diagnosis can be confirmed by electromyography of the levator ani muscle, which will show the action potentials continuing loudly when there ought to be electrical silence (see p. 143). Sometimes listening to the noise of the action potentials on a loudspeaker enables the patient to inhibit them herself—biofeedback.

SPHINCTER DAMAGE

I Prostatectomy. The bladder neck is removed as an integral part of the operation of transurethral resection for benign enlargement of the prostate (see p. 199)

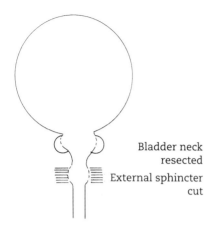

Fig. 17.13 Incontinence following division of both sphincters.

Bladder neck resected
External sphincter cut

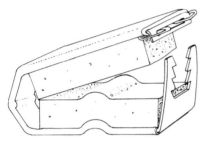

Fig. 17.14 Cunningham clamp.

and radical prostatectomy for cancer (see p. 211). Sometimes the supramembranous component of the external sphincter is cut by accident during transurethral resection (see p. 199) (Fig. 17.13).

2   Fractured pelvis. The sphincters may be injured if the bladder neck is lacerated by a fracture of the pelvis, or if the presacral sympathetic nerves are torn.

3   Cancer of the prostate. Prostatic cancer may infiltrate the sphincters causing them to lie permanently stiff and half-open.

Investigation of these patients will show a normal, stable detrusor, but negligible outflow resistance. Treatment is difficult: when the lesion is minor, the external sphincter may be strengthened by pelvic floor exercises. In more serious cases an appliance is used to compress the urethra. The oldest is the Cunningham clip (Fig. 17.14), whose sponge–rubber jaws gently compress the urethra. It can be put on and off by the patient, is cheap and relatively safe.

The newest is the Brantley–Scott artificial sphincter. A thin silicone balloon shaped like a doughnut is placed round the urethra and connected to a reservoir which can be emptied or filled by a bulb placed under the skin where the patient can compress it. The device is a very expensive miracle of engineering, but being a foreign body, is apt to suffer mechanical failure, infection, and erosion into the urethra (Fig. 17.15).

HERNIATION OF THE BASE OF THE BLADDER THROUGH THE PELVIC FLOOR

In women there is a short length of urethra above the levator ani shelf. When she coughs, the abdominal pressure squeezes this length of urethra by exactly the same amount as it squeezes the bladder. In many women, especially but not always those who have borne children, the normal gap for the urethra is enlarged, allowing it to descend below the levator ani, so that the intra-abdominal pressure can no longer squeeze it shut (Fig. 17.16). When the patient coughs or laughs there is a little spurt of urine—stress incontinence.

Because a very similar escape of urine is seen in detrusor instability (see above) patients who present with this symptom need urodynamic testing to rule out detrusor instability, before they are accepted as having genuine stress incontinence (GSI).

Clinical examination in GSI will show leakage of urine when the patient coughs, and it can be prevented by lifting up the anterior wall of the vagina with a finger on either side of the urethra (Bonney's or Marshall's test). The test should be done with the patient standing upright (Fig. 17.17).

Treatment of Genuine Stress Incontinence (GSI)

There are five procedures as follows.

1   Stamey, Raz, Pereira sutures. Described by various surgeons, non-absorbable sutures are placed to lift up the vaginal wall on either side of the urethra, just as in

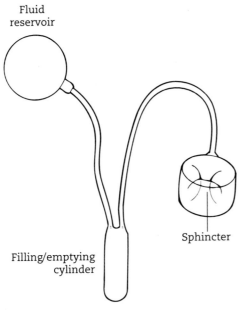

Fluid reservoir

Filling/emptying cylinder

Sphincter

Fig. 17.15 Brantley–Scott artificial sphincter.

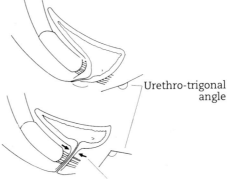

Urethro-trigonal angle

Intra-abdominal pressure

Fig. 17.16 Herniation of the bladder through the pelvic floor: the aim of all operations is to lift the urethra up again so that any increase of intra-abdominal pressure will compress the urethra.

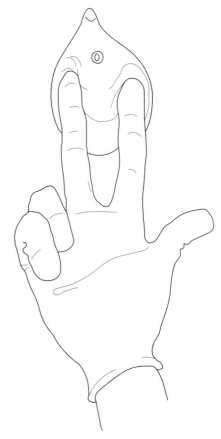

Fig. 17.17 Marshall's test.

the Bonney–Marshall clinical test (see p. 187) (Fig. 17.18). The operation is very easy for the patient, but the stitches tend to cut out like cheesewire and there is a high recurrence rate after 2 years.

2 Anterior colporrhaphy. Through a vaginal incision the connective tissue on either side of the urethra is approximated to support the neck of the bladder. The long-term results are discouraging (Fig. 17.19).

3 Vaginal colposuspension (Marshall–Marchetti–Krantz, MMK, or Burch operation). This is the classical and most reliable procedure, which has been 'invented' by several surgeons. Essentially, stitches are placed into the vaginal wall on either side of the urethra, and then through the periosteum of the pubis (MMK) or the

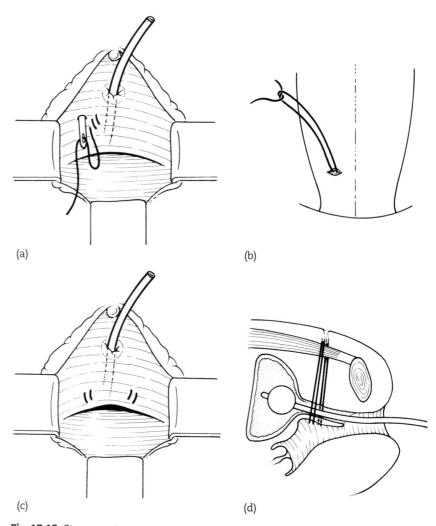

(a)

(b)

(c)

(d)

Fig. 17.18 Stamey sutures.

pectineal fascia (Burch). The end result is to achieve something comparable to the Marshall–Bonney test (Fig. 17.20).

4 Sling operations (Millin's sling). Another rediscovered procedure which involves a sling of some convenient material, preferably living rather than artificial, that is used to lift up the bladder neck on a hammock. Millin used a strip of rectus abdominis fascia. Others have tried different artificial materials, but they tend eventually to erode like cheesewire into the bladder and form a stone (Fig. 17.21).

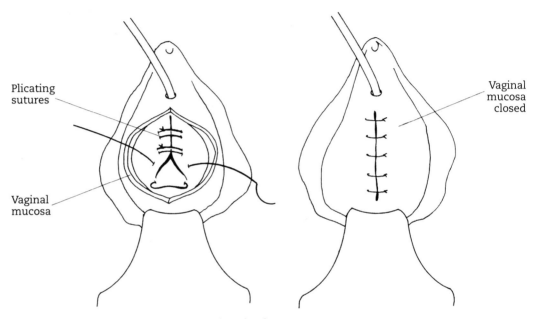

Plicating sutures

Vaginal mucosa

Vaginal mucosa closed

Fig. 17.19 Anterior colporrhaphy.

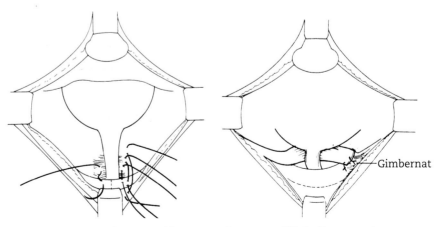

Fig. 17.20 Vaginal colposuspension.

Gimbernat

Fig. 17.21 Millin's sling operation.

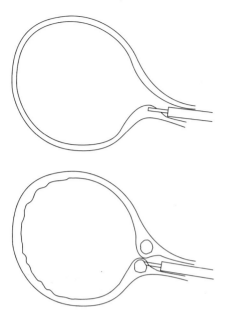

Fig. 17.22 Injections of Teflon or collagen paste around the bladder neck.

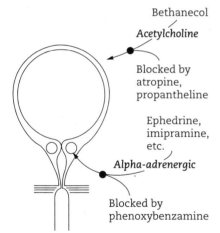

Fig. 17.23 Action of drugs on the bladder.

5 Periurethral injections. Various substances have been injected around the bladder neck for incontinence. A suspension of Teflon was the first, but was given up when it was found to migrate into the brain of experimental animals. Collagen paste is commonly used, and suspensions of the patient's own fat are now under trial. These substances give bulk to the tissue around the bladder neck or sphincter (Fig. 17.22).

PHARMACOLOGICAL TREATMENT

Medication seldom does any good in the common disorders of bladder function. The smooth muscle of the bladder is usually regarded as cholinergic, that of the sphincters as α-adrenergic (Fig. 17.23). To encourage the bladder to empty one can give bethanecol to release acetylcholine from the postganglionic fibres in the detrusor, and to discourage an overactive detrusor, give propantheline to block this action. These drugs seldom work on the detrusor that is exhausted by obstruction or rendered unstable from whatever cause.

Weakness of the smooth muscle of the sphincters is occasionally helped by an adrenergic drug such as ephedrine or imipramine, and α-blockers are sometimes effective in treating detrusor sphincter dyssynergia (see p. 199).

FURTHER READING

Abrams P, Blaivas JG, Stanton SL, Andersen JT (1988) The standardisation of terminology of lower urinary tract function. *Scand J Urol Nephrol* **114**: 5.

Burch JC (1961) Urethrovaginal fixation to Cooper's ligament for correction of stress incontinence, cystocele and prolapse. *Am J Obstet Gynecol* **81**, 281–90.

Chandiramani VA, Peterson T, Duthie GS, Fowler CJ (1996) Urodynamic changes during therapeutic intravesical instillations of capsaicin. *Br J Urol* **77**: 92.

Eckford SD, Jackson SR, Lewis PA, Abrams P (1996) The continence control pad—a new external urethral occlusion device in the management of stress incontinence. *Br J Urol* **77**: 538.

Hahn I, Milsom I (1996) Treatment of female stress urinary incontinence with a new anatomically shaped vaginal device (Conveen Continence Guard). *Br J Urol* **77**: 711.

Malone-Lee J (1996) Enuresis. *Curr Op Urol* **6**: 189–91.

Marshall VF, Marchetti AA, Krantz KE (1949) The correction of stress incontinence by simple vesico-urethral suspension. *Surg Gynecol Obstet* **88**: 509.

Mills R, Persad R, Ashken MH (1996) Long-term results with the Stamey operation for stress incontinence of urine. *Br J Urol* **77**: 86.

Mundy AR (1993) *Urodynamic and Reconstructive Surgery of the Lower Urinary Tract.* Edinburgh, Churchill Livingstone.

Sheriff MKM, Shah PJR, Fowler C, Mundy AR, Craggs MD (1996) Neuromodulation of detrusor hyper-reflexia by functional magnetic stimulation of the sacral roots. *Br J Urol* **78**: 39.

Woo HH, Rosario DJ, Chapple CR (1995) Stone formation on permanent suture material used previously in colposuspension. *Br J Urol* **76**: 139.

Yeung CK, Godley ML, Ho CKW *et al.* (1995) Some new insights into bladder function in infancy. *Br J Urol* **76**: 235.

Bethanecol

Acetylcholine

Blocked by atropine, propantheline

Ephedrine, imipramine, etc.

Alpha-adrenergic

Blocked by phenoxybenzamine

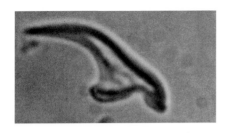

The Prostate Gland: Benign Disorders

SURGICAL ANATOMY

The prostate is made up of two zones which fit into each other like an egg in an egg-cup. Benign enlargement mainly arises in the inner zone, cancer in the outer. The ejaculatory ducts run between the two zones and empty into the urethra at the verumontanum (Fig. 18.1).

The prostate is closely related to the three elements of the sphincter in the male.

I The bladder neck, internal sphincter, is a collection of α-adrenergic smooth muscle, supplied by sympathetic nerve fibres.

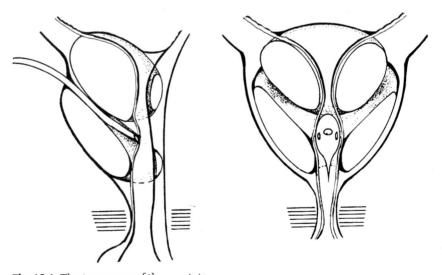

Fig. 18.1 The two zones of the prostate.

2   The supramembranous external sphincter, partly smooth muscle, partly striated, is just below the verumontanum, supplied by sympathetic nerve fibres.

3   The levator ani, voluntary striated muscle supplied by the pudendal nerve.

ANATOMICAL RELATIONS

Anteriorly is the symphysis pubis. Posteriorly the prostate is separated from the rectum by the fascia of Denonvilliers. Behind and above the prostate lie the bladder, seminal vesicles, vasa deferentia and ureters (Fig. 18.2).

STRUCTURE OF THE PROSTATE

The prostate is made up of glandular tubules which open into the back of the urethra. The contents of each tubule are squeezed out by a contractile sleeve of smooth muscle. Tubules and muscle are supported by a stroma of connective

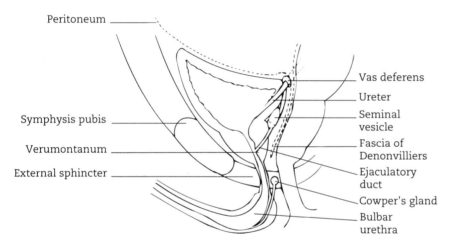

Fig. 18.2 Surgical anatomy of the prostate.

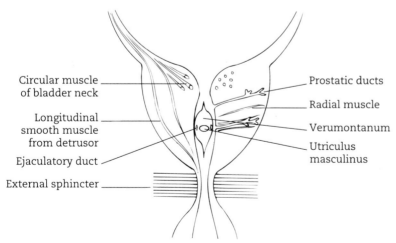

Fig. 18.3 Structure of the prostate.

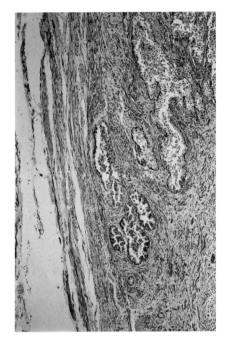

Fig. 18.4 Section through the edge of the prostate showing how the connective tissue of the 'capsule' is continuous with that surrounding the vessels outside. Courtesy of Mr Basil Page.

tissue. The three elements of the prostate, glands, muscle and stroma, can all enlarge and shrink at different times of life (Fig. 18.3).

In childhood there are very few glands: they appear and develop in puberty. In old age hypertrophy of one or all three elements, glands, muscle and stroma, gives rise to the nodules of benign prostatic enlargement. These nodules may compress the outer zone of the prostate into a thin shell and deform the prostate so as to give the appearance of having two 'lateral lobes' and one 'middle lobe'. These 'lobes' are not true functional entities as in the lung or the liver, but artefacts caused by the way the prostate is confined by the symphysis and the bladder.

Unlike many other abdominal organs, the prostate does not have a thick tough capsule, but only a thin film of connective tissue separates the surrounding fat and veins from the glandular tissue of the outer zone. This is important, because the concept of the 'capsule' is repeatedly referred to in discussions on the surgery of the prostate, nearly always incorrectly (Fig. 18.4).

PHYSIOLOGY

During ejaculation it is thought that the prostate contracts to secrete about 0.5 ml of fluid which is added to the ejaculate: but this is not certain nor does anyone know what the prostatic secretion is then supposed to do—it is presumed to play some role in the function of the semen, but most of what is written about the topic is pure guesswork.

INFLAMMATION OF THE PROSTATE

Acute prostatitis

Obstruction downstream to the prostate may force urine up into its ducts which, if infected, causes inflammation. Blood-borne infection is equally common. Whatever the route of the infection, the prostate becomes enlarged, painful on rectal palpation, and may cause painful and obstructed micturition. Pathogens may be recovered from the urine. Colour Doppler transrectal ultrasound scanning may show hyperaemia (Fig. 18.5).

Treatment requires an antibiotic that can reach the alkaline milieu of the prostate, e.g. trimethoprim, erythromycin or cinoxacin. A good combination is a short course of cinoxacin in the acute attack, followed by 4–6 weeks of a low dose of trimethoprim.

In most cases acute prostatitis resolves completely. Very rarely there is suppuration and an abscess forms which is best drained transurethrally, before it bursts spontaneously into the rectum (Fig. 18.6).

Acute prostatitis is a disorder which may relapse without warning.

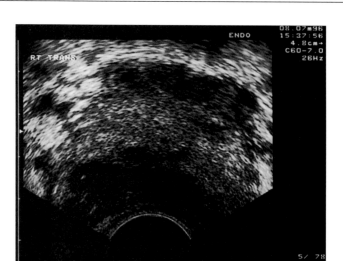

Fig. 18.5 Transrectal Doppler scan showing hyperaemia in a case of acute prostatitis.

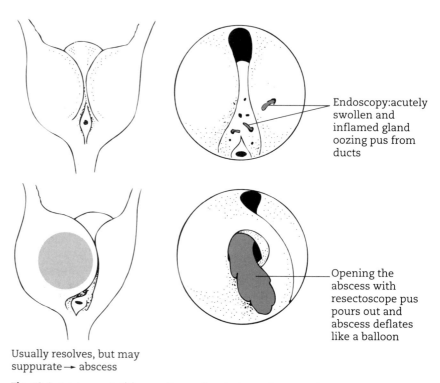

Endoscopy: acutely swollen and inflamed gland oozing pus from ducts

Opening the abscess with resectoscope pus pours out and abscess deflates like a balloon

Usually resolves, but may suppurate → abscess

Fig. 18.6 Acute prostatitis usually resolves but may form an abscess.

Chronic bacterial prostatitis

Persistent discomfort in the perineum with painful micturition is often attributed to chronic prostatitis. To prove it urine is collected in two parts (VB1 and VB2). Then the prostate is massaged transrectally to express fluid, which is collected (EPS). Finally a third urine specimen is collected (VB3). A diagnosis of infection in the prostate is made if the colony count (see p. 13) of bacteria in EPS and VB3 is greater than in VB1 and VB2.

The organisms that are recovered may be the usual *Escherichia coli* but *Chlamydia trachomatis* and *Trichomonas vaginalis* are found from time to time but their detection requires special culture techniques.

TREATMENT
The principles of the treatment of chronic bacterial prostatitis are the same as for any persistent bacterial infection, with the added difficulty that in the prostate the milieu is alkaline and many of the standard antibiotics do not penetrate the gland. For *Chlamydia* tetracyclines are usually effective, and for *Trichomonas* a week's course of metronidazole is given.

Prostatodynia

For each patient in whom bacterial infection can be proven there are dozens who complain of vague pain in the perineum, discomfort on voiding and sexual inadequacy. Usually there is a psychosexual problem, made worse when they are told that they have chronic prostatitis, especially if this must be treated by a course of 'prostatic massage', a treatment which is as uncomfortable as it is irrational—no other inflammation is made better by being forcibly squeezed.

In the absence of any scientific explanation for it, the treatment is necessarily unsatisfactory. The important thing is not to make it worse by futile or meddlesome intervention. Sympathy and the provision of analgesia, e.g. with diclofenac suppositories, often brings about symptomatic relief. Unfortunately prostatodynia is an entity which lends itself to quackery (see prostatic hyperthermia, below).

BENIGN ENLARGEMENT OF THE PROSTATE

AETIOLOGY
Over the age of 40 all men have nodular hyperplasia in the prostate but only one in 10 develop obstruction that needs treatment. Size is irrelevant: the smallest prostates may cause severe obstruction: huge glands none at all. The cause is not known although there is endless speculation as to some imbalance between

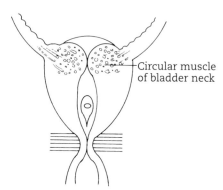

Fig. 18.7 Hypertrophy of the smooth muscle of the bladder neck.

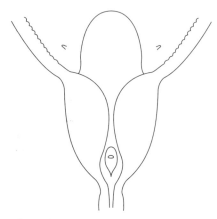

Fig. 18.8 The middle 'lobe' may protrude into the bladder.

oestrogens and androgens which is largely based on animal experiments of doubtful relevance in humans.

PATHOLOGY

Three factors act to cause obstruction as follows.

1 Smooth muscle. The α-adrenergic smooth muscle fibres in the prostate, especially around the bladder neck, fail to relax as the detrusor contracts (see p. 185). This is sometimes accompanied by hypertrophy of the smooth muscle (Fig. 18.7) and endoscopy may show a tight ring at the bladder neck without enlargement of the prostate.

2 Adenoma. A more or less large bulge of any or all three 'lobes' of the prostate may obstruct the lumen. The middle lobe alone may protrude like a thumb into the bladder (Fig. 18.8). The inner zone of the prostate enlarges and the outer zone is compressed into a shell, often incorrectly called the 'capsule', while the verumontanum is displaced down towards the external sphincter (Fig. 18.9).

3 Detrusor failure. The response of the detrusor to obstruction is described on p. 184. In the first phase it becomes stronger and more jumpy. Later it becomes weaker and less forcible, and this weakness is often an additional factor contributing to the development of further obstruction. Detrusor failure may occur gradually, or suddenly.

(a) Acute detrusor failure may be precipitated by some other unrelated illness, e.g. a heart attack or confinement to bed for an operation on some other system, and causes acute retention of urine. This is very painful. The bladder is felt as a hard suprapubic mass. Often all that is necessary is to let the urine out with a catheter and normal voiding will be resumed.

(b) In chronic detrusor failure there is no pain. The big distended bladder is often soft and difficult to feel. A little urine escapes from time to time—overflow incontinence (see p. 185) (Fig. 18.10).

(c) In practice there is a third very common category: these are men who have had a long crescendo of progressive obstruction and then suddenly develop acute retention. This is sometimes referred to as acute-on-chronic retention.

Complications of obstruction

1 Changes in the detrusor. If the obstruction is not relieved, the detrusor will develop trabeculation, sacculation and form diverticula. Eventually it loses the power to contract, which may be irreversible.

2 Complications from residual urine. Infection and stone formation are apt to occur whenever there is a large pocket of stagnant urine (see p. 75).

3 Obstructive uropathy. Neglected obstruction leads to loss of renal tubular

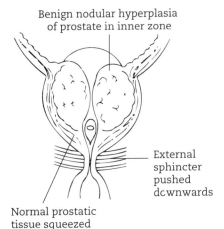

Benign nodular hyperplasia of prostate in inner zone

External sphincter pushed downwards

Normal prostatic tissue squeezed out into 'capsule'

Fig. 18.9 Formation of bulky adenomas in the prostate.

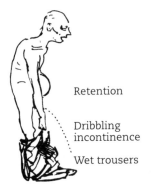

Retention

Dribbling incontinence

Wet trousers

Fig. 18.10 Overflow incontinence.

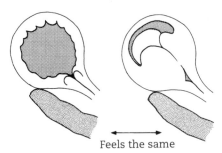

Feels the same

Fig. 18.11 The finger in the rectum cannot distinguish urine under pressure in the bladder from a big prostate.

function, the inability to conserve water or salt, and ultimately to impaired glomerular filtration leading to uraemia (see pp. 52 and 114).

The objectives of the management of benign enlargement of the prostate are quite simple, to diagnose and relieve obstruction before any of these three types of complication have occurred.

Diagnosis of prostatic obstruction

HISTORY
The symptoms that bring the patient to the doctor before the patient has developed complications are usually frequency of micturition and a poor flow, but these are not specific, and every patient requires a careful history. In many centres the patient is asked to complete a questionnaire, from which a 'symptom score' can be calculated. This should never be a substitute for listening to the patient carefully, especially since these symptom scores have been shown to be the same in men and women, and not to correlate at all with objective evidence of obstruction.

PHYSICAL SIGNS
Abdominal palpation may reveal a chronically obstructed bladder (see p. 3) but this is a late feature of the disease. Rectal examination cannot distinguish between a tight bladder full of residual urine and a large prostatic adenoma (Fig. 18.11), nor can it feel a middle lobe that sticks up into the bladder out of reach of the finger (Fig. 18.12).

INVESTIGATIONS
1 Flow rate. Flow rates vary from day to day, and a poor flow may not necessarily mean obstruction: it may result from a weak detrusor. If the detrusor has undergone considerable hypertrophy it can compensate for obstruction and produce a good flow rate. Nevertheless an impaired flow rate less than 10 ml/s is a significant part of the clinical pattern (Fig. 18.13).
2 Residual urine. The residual urine can be measured by abdominal ultrasound. Again this may vary from day to day. The abdominal ultrasound can detect dilatation of the ureters and renal pelves and will reveal gross trabeculation and diverticula (Fig. 18.14).
3 Transrectal ultrasound. The volume of the prostate can be measured from the ultrasound image, but since volume has little relationship to obstruction, transrectal ultrasound is really not relevant. It is, however, often performed in the hope of detecting prostatic cancer (see p. 15) (Fig. 18.15).
4 Urodynamic studies. The only way of making certain that there is outflow obstruction to the bladder is by means of a comprehensive urodynamic investigation (see p. 142) which must include the measurement of the pressure inside the

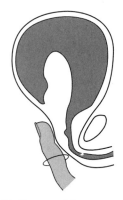

Fig. 18.12 The rectal finger cannot feel a large middle lobe.

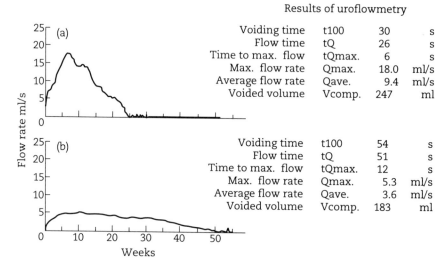

Results of uroflowmetry

(a)

Voiding time	t100	30	s
Flow time	tQ	26	s
Time to max. flow	tQmax.	6	s
Max. flow rate	Qmax.	18.0	ml/s
Average flow rate	Qave.	9.4	ml/s
Voided volume	Vcomp.	247	ml

(b)

Voiding time	t100	54	s
Flow time	tQ	51	s
Time to max. flow	tQmax.	12	s
Max. flow rate	Qmax.	5.3	ml/s
Average flow rate	Qave.	3.6	ml/s
Voided volume	Vcomp.	183	ml

Fig. 18.13 Urine flow rates in (a) normal, and (b) benign enlargement of the prostate.

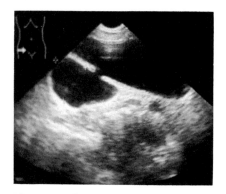

Fig. 18.14 Ultrasound after trying to empty the bladder showing large residual as well as a diverticulum.

bladder during micturition. Since, to be accurate, this involves inserting a fine suprapubic catheter the test is not done as a routine investigation, except when there is real doubt about the diagnosis, usually in younger patients whose main complaint is of frequency.

DIFFERENTIAL DIAGNOSIS

1   Cancer. The symptoms of bladder cancer may so closely mimic prostatism that every elderly man complaining of frequency and so on should have his urine examined for red cells and cancer cells (see p. 11).

2   Stricture. The symptoms of obstruction by enlargement of the prostate are identical to obstruction from a urethral stricture, so that if there is, for example, a history of previous cardiac surgery (when a catheter would have been passed) or some other urethral instrumentation, the diagnosis of stricture should be considered (see p. 233).

3   Neuropathy. Neuropathic lesions, especially a central lumbar disc protrusion, can mimic prostatism (see p. 178).

4   Polyuria. The alteration in the excretion of the pituitary antidiuretic hormone that occurs in old age and in mild heart failure causes nocturnal urinary frequency which has nothing to do with the prostate (see p. 35).

5   Depression. Many a sad old widower wakes in the small hours because he is lonely and depressed. He goes to the toilet, but cannot get back to sleep. So he gets up and makes a cup of tea. Then he must urinate again, and so on. The patient will tell you the diagnosis if you only listen.

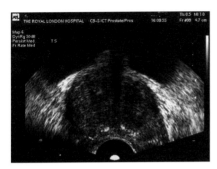

Fig. 18.15 Transrectal ultrasound images showing enlargement of the prostate.

Treatment

Wait and see

Many elderly men go through a year or two during which their prostate irritates them, but not very severely, and then it gets better without any treatment (or if they are given a placebo in the course of a clinical trial). They may still have to urinate once or twice in the night, but their daytime activities are unaffected. They have a reasonable flow rate and their residual urine is negligible. Suggest he comes back and reports progress in 6 months or so.

α-blockers

When the prostate is small and the patient's symptoms dominated by frequency, the problem may be a mild form of detrusor–sphincter dyssynergia (see p. 185) and an α-blocker, e.g. indoramine or prazosin, often relieves symptoms.

Finasteride

Finasteride prevents a hydrogen atom being added to testosterone to activate it inside the prostate cell, and may shrink the glandular part of the prostate and bring about a small improvement in flow rate and residual urine. It makes the prostatic specific antigen level fall, and in many patients appears to relieve symptoms, and seems to do no harm. It is a useful variant on the wait and see approach.

Surgery

Open prostatectomy. Around 1890 it was found almost by accident that the adenoma in the inner zone could be enucleated from the compressed shell of outer zone with a finger. In the early days this was performed via a suprapubic incision into the bladder, or through a perineal incision. In 1943 Millin developed the retropubic approach which is still used for very large glands (Fig. 18.16).

Transurethral resection. Improved technology made it possible to remove the inner zone adenoma with a telescope passed along the urethra (Fig. 18.17). This operation, which is usually performed under televisual control, carries an operative mortality of less than 1%, but there are still complications.

1 Bleeding can be severe during the operation.

2 Stricture develops in the urethra afterwards in about 3% of men.

3 Because the bladder neck is removed along with the prostate there is retrograde ejaculation of semen.

4 Impotence occurs in 10–15% after prostatectomy.

5 Incontinence of urine may be the result of a technical mistake whereby the supramembranous external sphincter is injured, or may be due to persistent detrusor instability. It is one reason for being cautious in men who have frequency as their presenting feature.

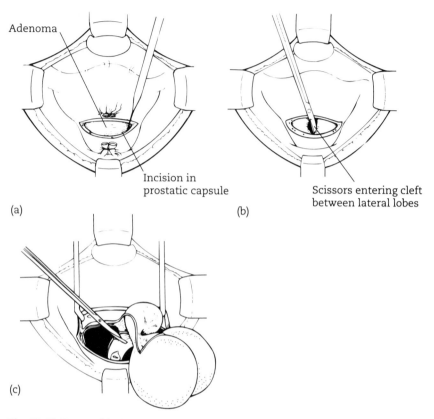

Adenoma

Incision in
prostatic capsule

(a)

Scissors entering cleft
between lateral lobes

(b)

(c)

Fig. 18.16 Retropubic prostatectomy.

Transurethral prostatectomy

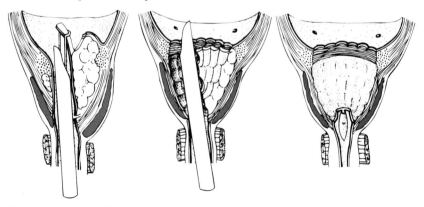

Fig. 18.17 Transurethral resection of the prostate.

Transurethral incision of the prostate. Instead of removing the inner zone, an incision is made through the bladder neck and prostate (see Fig. 18.18). There is less bleeding and a shorter hospital stay. No tissue is removed for histological diagnosis and the long-term results are still uncertain.

Transurethral vaporization of the prostate. The prostatic tissue can be coagulated or vaporized by a special diathermy current or a laser (Fig. 18.19). The method appears to remove the inner zone tissue in a way that is comparable to transurethral resection but the long-term complication rate and results are still unknown.

Thermocoagulation. The last decade has seen the introduction of many new devices which cook the adenoma by means of high frequency energy provided from a transmitter in the urethra, lasers or needles inserted into the prostate (Fig. 18.20). The enthusiasm with which these gadgets have been publicized has far exceeded the evidence that they are effective or safe, and has often relied upon symptom scores (see p. 197).

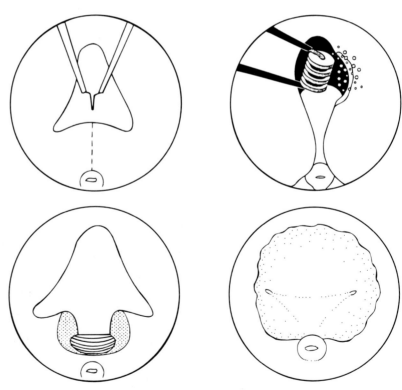

Fig. 18.18 Transurethral incision of the prostate.

Fig. 18.19 Transurethral vaporization of the prostate using diathermy.

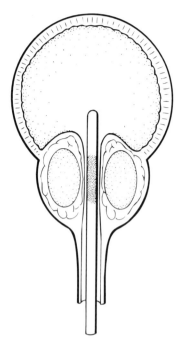

Fig. 18.20 Transurethral hyperthermia of the prostate.

Freezing. The inner zone adenoma can be frozen, leaving necrotic tissue which is slowly phagocytosed. This method enjoyed popularity 30 years ago, and has recently been reinvented.

PRACTICAL MANAGEMENT OF PROSTATIC DISORDERS

Acute retention of urine
When this follows some other illness, e.g. a recent heart attack or an operation to replace the hip, the bladder is emptied with a catheter which is left in position until the patient is up and about.

Acute-on-chronic retention
When acute retention develops after a long crescendo of prostatic symptoms the catheter is left in, and arrangements are made for prostatectomy as soon as possible. The patient can safely go home during this interval.

Chronic retention
This is an entirely different entity because (i) the detrusor is often badly damaged, and (ii) there may be severe impairment of renal function with dehydration, salt-depletion and anaemia. If the creatinine is elevated you may be sure the patient is also dehydrated, etc.

After the bladder is emptied, there may be a profuse postobstructive diuresis during which such a large volume of fluid is lost that the patient may become shocked. Intravenous saline may be needed to make up the deficiency in extracellular volume. Fortunately the renal tubules usually recover, but during this time anaemia may require transfusion, heart failure may require treatment, and the mental condition of the patient may need care. The old man is sick, frightened, confused and fuddled by medication. He needs kind voices to talk to, plenty of light, company and stimulation. The last things he needs are isolation and sedation. There is no company he needs so much as that of his family and friends. A little alcohol, within reason, may comfort him: it never did the kidneys any harm whatever it might have done to his liver.

Preparations for prostatectomy

1   Consent. Whatever technique is used, retrograde ejaculation is likely to occur and must be explained. The younger man who might still wish to have children might want to weigh this in the balance against the risks of putting off the removal of the obstruction. At any age the risks of ejaculatory impotence must be explained.

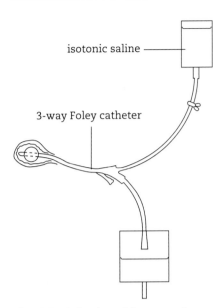

isotonic saline

3-way Foley catheter

Fig. 18.21 Irrigation of the prostatic fossa with a three-way catheter.

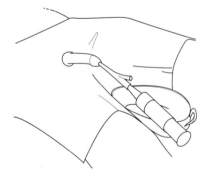

Fig. 18.22 Irrigation of the catheter with a bladder syringe.

2 Blood loss. After open or transurethral resection loss of blood can be sudden, unpredictable and occasionally life-threatening. Blood should always be grouped and if the gland is known to be very large, two to three units should be cross-matched.

3 Antibiotics. If there is known infection, or if a catheter has been in position, then antibiotics are always given to protect against septicaemia. It is still a matter of debate whether they are needed in every cold operation.

Postoperative care

The catheter
After all forms of prostatectomy a catheter is left in the bladder, usually a three-way catheter which allows saline to run in and out of the bladder to dilute blood and prevent clots from blocking the catheter (Fig. 18.21). Some surgeons rely on natural formation of urine to irrigate the bladder, and encourage this with a diuretic.

If a chip of prostate or a blood clot does block the catheter an attempt is made to wash it out with a bladder syringe (Fig. 18.22) using strict aseptic precautions. If this fails the catheter is removed and a new one is passed.

Reactionary haemorrhage
Reactionary haemorrhage may occur after any type of prostatectomy. The bladder fills with blood clot which cannot be evacuated with a bladder syringe. The patient is returned at once to the operating theatre where the clot is removed with an Ellik evacuator and the offending vessels coagulated. Very occasionally the reactionary bleeding can be so furious that the only way to stop it is to open the retropubic space and pack the prostatic fossa.

Removal of the catheter
All the bleeding has usually stopped within 24–48 h, and the catheter is removed. At first there may be some discomfort on passing urine, and an occasional leak if the patient coughs or strains. This soon recovers.

Going home
Patients usually go home after 4 or 5 days, but the empty cavity from which the inner zone tissue has been removed is still raw and unhealed, and secondary haemorrhage may occur at any moment. It makes sense to advise him to avoid strain: a good rule is to do anything he ordinarily can do in his carpet slippers. Around the 10th postoperative day there is often a little haematuria, and patients understand if it is explained beforehand that it may bleed a little when the 'scab' comes away. Very rarely the patient must be readmitted to have clot irrigated out of the bladder.

Recovery

Recovery is not complete until the prostatic fossa has been completely relined with urothelium and this may take about 6 weeks. Until then the patient will notice some frequency and urgency, and the urine will continue to be a little cloudy, raising the suggestion of infection. Antibiotics are not needed, however, unless there is a significant growth of bacteria.

FURTHER READING

Caine M (1995) Reflections on α-blockade the rapy for benign prostatic hyperplasia. *Br J Urol* **75**: 265.

Dunsmuir WD, Emberton M (1996) There is significant sexual dysfunction following TURP. *Br J Urol* **77**: suppl. 39.

Emberton M, Neal DE, Black N *et al.* (1996) The effect of prostatectomy on symptom severity and quality of life. *Br J Urol* **77**: 233.

Feneley MR, Gillatt DA, Hehir M, Kirby RS (1996) A review of radical prostatectomy from three centres in the UK: clinical presentation and outcome. *Br J Urol* **78**: 911.

Freyer PJ (1901) Total extirpation of the prostate for radical cure of enlargement of that organ. *Br Med J* i: 125.

Hall JC, Christiansen KJ, England P *et al.* (1996) Antibiotic prophylaxis for patients undergoing transurethral resection of the prostate. *Urology* **47**: 852.

Hargreave TB, Heynes CF, Kendrick SW, Whyte B, Clarke JA (1996) Mortality after transurethral and open prostatectomy in Scotland. *Br J Urol* **77**: 547.

Hines JEW (1996) Symptom indices in bladder outlet obstruction. *Br J Urol* **77**: 494.

Hofner K, Jonas U (1996) Urodynamics in benign prostatic hyperplasia. *Curr Op Urol* **6**: 184.

McGregor R, Dawkins G, Thilagarajah R, Anson K, Miller R (1996) Laser prostatectomy: 3 years follow-up, a cause for concern. *Br J Urol* **77**: suppl. 9 (43).

Meade WMN, Mcloughlin MG (1996) Endoscopic roller-ball electrovaporization of the prostate—the sandwich technique: evaluation of the initial efficacy and morbidity in the treatment of benign prostatic obstruction. *Br J Urol* **77**: 696.

Millin T (1947) *Retropubic Urinary Surgery.* Edinburgh, Churchill Livingstone.

Orandi A (1985) Transurethral incision of prostate—645 cases in 15 years. A chronological appraisal. *Br J Urol* **57**: 703.

Medical Research Council (MRC) Prostate Cancer Working Party (1997) Immediate versus deferred treatment for advanced prostatic cancer: initial results of the Medical Research Council trial. *Br J Urol* **79**: 235.

Nakamura S, Kobayshi Y, Tozuka K, Tukkue A, Kimura A, Hamada C (1996) Circadian changes in urine volume and frequency in elderly men. *J Urol* **156**: 1275.

Sattar AA, Noel C, Vanderhaeghen JJ, Schulman CC, Wespes E (1995) Prostate capsule: computerized morphometric analysis of its components. *Urology* **46**: 178.

Squires B, Gillatt DA (1995) Massive bladder calculus as a complication of a titanium prostatic stent. *Br J Urol* **75**: 252.

Stoner E (1992) The clinical effects of a 5-alpha reductase inhibitor—finasteride—on benign prostatic hyperplasia. *J Urol* **147**: 1298.

Veneziano S, Pavlica P, Mannini D (1995) Color Doppler ultrasonographic scanning in prostatitis: clinical correlation. *Eur Urol* **28**: 6.

Venn SN, Montgomery BS, Sheppard S, Lloyd-Davies RW, Tiptaft RC (1995) Microwave hyperthermia in benign prostatic hypertrophy: a controlled clinical trial. *Br J Urol* **76**: 73.

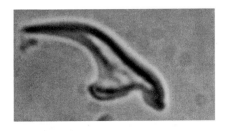

Prostate Cancer

AETIOLOGY

There are unexplained differences in the incidence of cancer of the prostate in different parts of the world: it is relatively uncommon in men of Japanese and Indian ancestry, and more common in those of African ancestry. The number of reported cases seems to be increasing, but this may be an artefact due to an increased interest, the growing number of elderly men who are surviving, and better ways of making the diagnosis.

INCIDENCE

At the age of 50 about 15% of prostates contain islands of cancer: by 80 the figure is nearly 100%. Cancer of the prostate accounts for less than 0.5% deaths in each age group over the age of 60, a proportion which has not changed in the last decades in Europe or the USA (Fig. 19.1). The total annual number of new cases shows an increase and this is frequently interpreted in an alarmist way to justify programmes of screening.

PATHOLOGY

Cancer usually arises in the outer zone which in elderly men is usually compressed into a shell by benign enlargement. Cancer does arise from the inner zone but seldom spreads and behaves as if it were almost benign (Fig. 19.2).

HISTOLOGICAL GRADE

The Gleason system is based on the assessment of the pattern of growth seen in two low power fields (Fig. 19.3), each assigned a number from 1 to 15, i.e. if well-

Fig. 19.1 In each age group the proportion of deaths from cancer of the prostate has not changed.

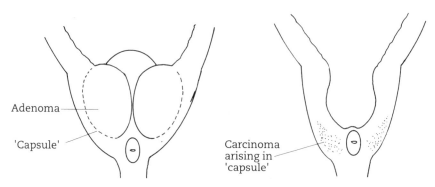

Fig. 19.2 Cancer arises in the outer zone of the prostate.

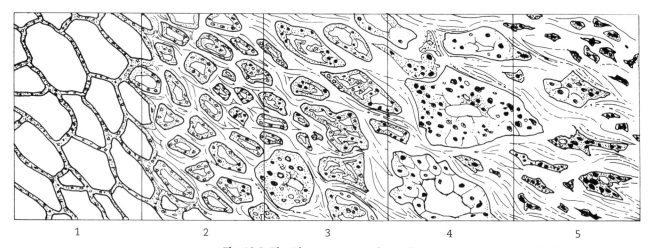

Fig. 19.3 The Gleason system: for each tumour two low power fields are assigned a score from 1 to 5: the Gleason score is the sum.

differentiated cancer is seen in both fields it may be given the Gleason grade 2 + 2 = 4 (Fig. 19.4). The World Health Organization (WHO) system recognizes three grades—G1, G2 and G3. The Gleason system correlates very well with the clinical behaviour of the tumour and its response to treatment.

TUMOUR MARKERS

Prostatic-specific antigen (PSA)

This is a protein secreted only by prostate cells whether benign or malignant. It spills over into the bloodstream where it can be measured, and it can be detected by immunofluorescent methods in histological sections.

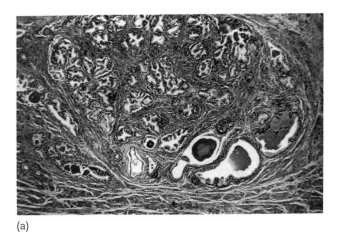

(a)

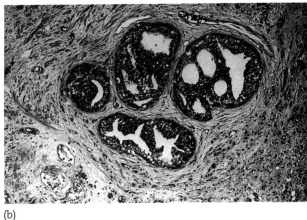

(b)

Fig. 19.4 (a) Benign hyperplasia. (b) Cancer—an area of Gleason 2 is surrounded by anaplastic Gleason 5.

Prostatic acid phosphatase

Prostate cells secrete a phosphatase which is active in an acid milieu. It can be measured by a biochemical or a more accurate radioimmunological assay. It has largely been superseded by the use of prostate-specific antigen (PSA).

STAGING OF PROSTATIC CANCER

Staging of prostate cancer takes into account its method of spread which is directly up into the bladder and seminal vesicles, but not through Denonvilliers' fascia into the rectum but instead grows around it to cause obstruction. It quickly invades the pelvic lymph nodes, and spreads by veins and lymphatics into the marrow of the lumbar spine, pelvis and femora. The TNM staging system is set out in Fig. 19.5.

CLINICAL FEATURES

PICKED UP BY SCREENING

Carcinoma of the prostate is often detected by chance with PSA. Knowing that little islands of cancer are present in most elderly men it is surprising that cancer is not discovered more often.

CHANCE FINDING AT TRANSURETHRAL REACTION OF THE PROSTATE

Carcinoma is found by chance in about 10% of patients undergoing transurethral resection of the prostate (TURP) for what was thought to be a benign enlarge-

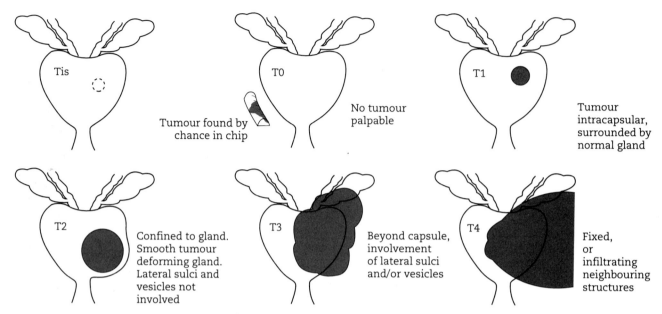

Fig. 19.5 TNM staging of prostatic cancer.

ment of the prostate. Knowing the true incidence of cancer in the prostate one would expect the figure to be higher, but of course TURP takes out mostly inner zone tissue, and spares the compressed outer zone in which most cancers arise.

LOCAL SYMPTOMS

Prostatism. Compression of the urethra may cause symptoms identical with those due to benign enlargement (see p. 197).

Rectal obstruction. If the cancer is encircling the rectum the patient may complain of pencil-thin stools and progressive constipation.

Uraemia. Ureteric obstruction may lead to hydroureter and hydronephrosis and, if bilateral, to uraemia.

DISTANT METASTASES

Metastases may occur anywhere, but usually involve the lumbar vertebrae, pelvis and femora to cause bone pain, a pathological fracture or spinal cord compression. These metastases are typically denser than the normal bone, i.e. osteoblastic

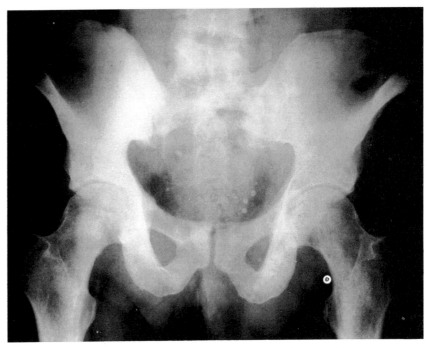

Fig. 19.6 X-ray of pelvis showing areas of increased density caused by metastases.

(Fig. 19.6). Occasionally fibrinolysins produced by metastases cause bruising and haemorrhages.

INVESTIGATIONS

TRANSRECTAL ULTRASOUND

The echogenicity of the prostate is determined by the amount of calcium in the tissues which in cancer may be greater or lesser than normal (Fig. 19.7). Any non-homogeneous area is biopsied using a Biopty or Trucut needle placed under ultrasonic control (Fig. 19.8). Several biopsies are taken from each side, and often show multifocal cancer. The ultrasound image may show that cancer has invaded the seminal vesicles or the periprostatic fat and so help to stage the case.

COMPUTED TOMOGRAPHY SCAN

The computed tomography (CT) scan may reveal enlarged pelvic lymph nodes and invasion of the seminal vesicles (Fig. 19.9).

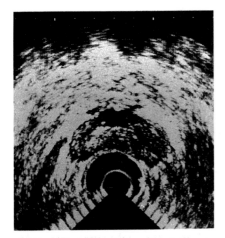

Fig. 19.7 Transrectal ultrasound showing cancer breaching the capsule on the left side.

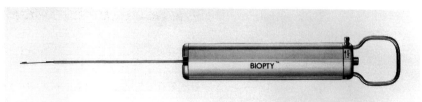

Fig. 19.8 Biopty needle for transrectal biopsy.

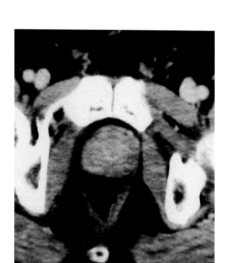

Fig. 19.9 CT scan showing carcinoma in the posterior right part of the prostate. Courtesy of Dr M.J. Kellett.

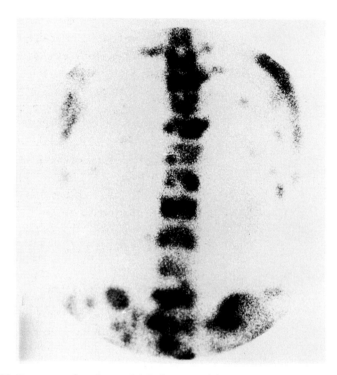

Fig. 19.11 Bone scan showing multiple 'hot spots' from metastases.

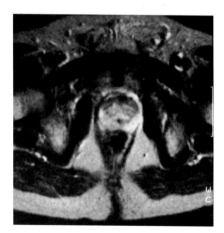

Fig. 19.10 MRI T2 weighted image showing loss of signal in the right peripheral zone. Courtesy of Dr Janet Husband.

MAGNETIC RESONANCE IMAGING

These images may be even more precise in staging the cancer and are often performed when radical prostatectomy is contemplated (Fig. 19.10).

BONE SCAN

The radionuclide ^{99m}Tc-MDP (methylene diphosphonate) is taken up by bone in proportion to the blood flow, so the increased vascularity of a metastasis shows as a 'hot spot' (Fig. 19.11). False positives are common from osteoarthritis and old fractures of the ribs. When the bones are very widely invaded there may be a 'superscan'.

TREATMENT

T0–T3—TUMOUR APPARENTLY CONFINED TO THE PROSTATE

There is a heated debate between those who favour radical prostatectomy for cancers that appear to be confined to the prostate, and those who favour surveillance—watchful waiting. The arguments in favour of radical surgery are:

1 More of those who survive for 10–15 years after radical surgery do so without residual cancer.

2 Radical prostatectomy avoids the misery of local recurrence in the pelvis.

3 If the operation is done correctly potency can be preserved so long as the cancer is not infiltrating the nerves to the penis, and incontinence is very rare.

The arguments against radical prostatectomy are:

1 Almost every elderly man has a small cancer in his prostate, but fewer than 0.5% die of it: 99.5% do not.

2 The only prospective controlled study to have been carried out showed no differences in survival after 20 years between men treated by radical surgery or surveillance.

3 Larger retrospective studies of Medicare patients show no difference in survival between those undergoing radical surgery and surveillance.

4 The morbidity of radical prostatectomy includes incontinence, stricture and impotence in a (debated but large) proportion of patients.

Radical prostatectomy

The prostate is approached through a lower abdominal incision. The lymph nodes along the internal iliac and obturator vessels are dissected and sent for frozen section, unless this has already been done by a laparoscopic procedure. The dorsal veins of the penis are doubly ligated and divided behind the symphysis, and the neurovascular bundles going to the penis are pushed aside out of harm's way (Fig. 19.12). The urethra is transected, and the prostate lifted up, to reveal the seminal vesicles, whose vessels are ligated. The bladder is then cut across at the level of the bladder neck, which is then narrowed, and sutured to the stump of the urethra over a catheter (Fig. 19.13).

STAGING LYMPH NODE DISSECTION

Most surgeons consider that radical prostatectomy is futile if the lymph nodes are involved and usually sample the lymph nodes around the obturator nerve and vessels before going ahead with radical surgery. This can be performed laparoscopically a few days before surgery is planned, or as the first stage of an open operation.

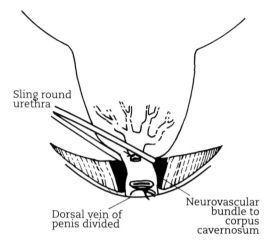

Fig. 19.12 Radical retropubic prostatectomy: the neurovascular bundles to the penis can be preserved.

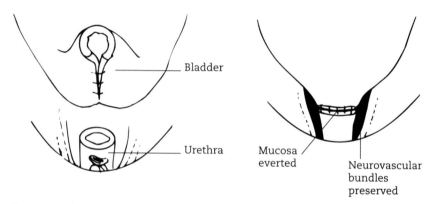

Fig. 19.13 After the prostate has been removed, the bladder is sutured to the stump of the urethra.

Radiotherapy

There is a third possibility, namely of irradiating the prostate using either external beam therapy with the linear accelerator, or inserting radioactive seeds into the prostate under transrectal ultrasound control.

No randomized prospective controlled study has ever shown that any type of radiation is better or worse than surveillance or radical prostatectomy. Survival is much the same, but residual cancer is found more often after radiation in the survivors than in those treated by surgery, even though it does not necessarily cause symptoms. Painful proctitis is a common early sequel of radiation, and impotence occurs in a proportion, probably as a result of radiation arteritis.

Involving the patient

In view of the considerable doubt that exists as to the choice of treatment the pros and cons of each different form of treatment should be explained so that an informed choice can be made. Some men find it repugnant to think that they might be walking around with cancer, and it does not help to point out that similar microscopic cancers occur in many other organs, e.g. kidney, lung and liver. Others find the prospect of incontinence and impotence no less undesirable and prefer to take their chance.

METASTASES

Malignant prostate cells start off by requiring a daily supply of testosterone without which they die. In cancer, mutant clones eventually emerge which no longer depend on testosterone, and this (on average) occurs in about 80% of men within 2 years of the diagnosis of metastases; however, among the 20% who do not develop metastases within 2 years there are many who survive for decades without any treatment.

Largely as a result of these and other anecdotal experiences, there was a feeling that no harm arose from deferring the treatment until metastases began to cause symptoms. This was the subject of a recent Medical Research Council controlled prospective trial, which showed an unacceptably high incidence of serious metastatic complications in patients for whom hormone therapy had been deferred.

Hormone therapy

The supply of testosterone can be cut off in a number of ways.

ORCHIECTOMY

The testicles may be removed, or a subcapsular orchiectomy may be performed which leaves something behind which feels like a normal testicle.

DIETHYLSTILBOESTROL

This is a synthetic oestrogen which blocks the products of metabolism of testosterone. Given in large doses of 5 mg/day it had a high incidence of cardiovascular side effects but a dose of 1 mg daily seems to be just as effective without cardiovascular sequelae.

LUTEINIZING HORMONE-RELEASING HORMONE AGONISTS

Zoladex and Leuprolide overstimulate the anterior pituitary gland until it is exhausted and can produce no more luteinizing hormone. As a result the testis and adrenal no longer secrete testosterone. However, during the first 2 weeks of treatment there is a sudden increase in the output of luteinizing hormone (LH) and a tide of testosterone, which may cause a 'flare-up' with pain and other complications from metastases, so LH-releasing hormone (LHRH) agonists are given in combination with drugs which block the action of testosterone in the cells — anti-androgens (see below).

5α-REDUCTASE INHIBITORS

5α-reductase inhibitors such as finasteride prevent the activation of testosterone to dihydrotestosterone but they are seldom used in the treatment of prostate cancer.

ANTI-ANDROGENS

Dihydrotestosterone acts on receptors in the cytosol of the prostate cell. These receptors are blocked by two types of anti-androgen: (i) steroids such as megestrol and cyproterone; and (ii) non-steroids such as flutamide, nilutamide and bicalutamide.

AROMATASE INHIBITORS

These prevent the action of aromatase, an enzyme in the prostate cell which converts adrenal steroids into testosterone. They are still under trial.

TOTAL ANDROGEN BLOCKADE

A combination of LHRH agonists given together with anti-androgens is claimed to give a small improvement (a matter of weeks) in survival but not everyone is convinced that this is justified by the side effects, let alone the expense of this additional therapy.

Radiotherapy

Isolated painful metastases respond dramatically to small doses of radiation, which can be particularly useful when there is a pathological fracture or spinal cord compression. Severe pain in the skeleton can be helped by hemi-body radiation, a technique in which one half of the body is irradiated, to control bony metastases. This also destroys the bone marrow in the irradiated bones, but after a few weeks to allow this marrow to be repopulated by haematogenous cells from the rest of the bone, the other half is irradiated.

Similar relief of pain can be produced by radioactive phosphorus-32, strontium-89 and diphosphonate.

Chemotherapy

So far, no combination of chemotherapy has been of any use in metastatic carcinoma of the prostate.

FURTHER READING

Arai Y, Kanamaru H, Moroi S et al. (1996) Radical prostatectomy for clinically localized prostate cancer: local tumor extension and prognosis. *Int J Urol* **3**: 373.

Barry MJ, Fleming C, Coley CM, Wasson JH, Fahs MC, Oesterling JE (1995) Should Medicare provide reimbursement for prostate-specific antigen testing for early detection of prostate cancer? Part IV: estimating the risks and benefits of an early detection program. *Urology* **46**: 445.

Barry MJ, Fleming C, Coley CM, Wasson JH, Fahs MC, Oesterling JE (1995) Should Medicare provide reimbursement for prostate-specific antigen testing for early detection of prostate cancer? Part III. Management strategies and outcomes. *Urology* **46**: 277.

Gil-Vernet JM (1996) Prostate cancer: anatomical and surgical considerations. *Br J Urol* **78**: 161.

Schroeder FH (1995) Screening, early detection, and treatment of prostate cancer: a European view. *Urology* **46**: (suppl. 3A), 62.

Zalcberg JR, Raghavan D, Marshall V, Thompson PJ (1996) Bilateral orchidectomy and flutamide versus orchidectomy alone in newly diagnosed patients with metastatic carcinoma of the prostate—an Australian multicentre trial. *Br J Urol* **77**: 865.

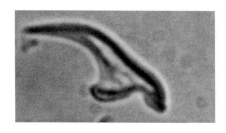

The Urethra

ANATOMY

In both sexes the urethra is lined with urothelium near the bladder and squamous epithelium near the external meatus. In between is modified columnar epithelium. Para-urethral glands enter all along the urethra, secreting mucus. Some of these glands are of special importance.

In males the most important para-urethral glands make up the prostate: in addition there is a pair of Cowper's glands in the levator ani, and a pair of Littré's glands near the external meatus. Any of these may become infected and form an abscess (Fig. 20.1).

The urethra is surrounded by the corpus spongiosum which in males expands to form the glans penis. Each corpus spongiosum is supported by a pair of corpora cavernosa, which are attached to the medial aspect of the ischiopubic rami (Fig. 20.2).

In females the urethra is shorter, and surrounded by a sleeve of erectile corpus spongiosum which continues into the glans of the clitoris, flanked by two smaller corpora cavernosa (Fig. 20.3).

SPHINCTERS

In males the three components of the sphincter surround the urethra at the bladder neck, the supramembranous sphincter and the levator ani (see p. 141).

In females there are the same three elements to the sphincter: the bladder neck: the intramural sleeve made up of a mixture of striated and smooth muscle, and below this the levator ani (Fig. 20.4).

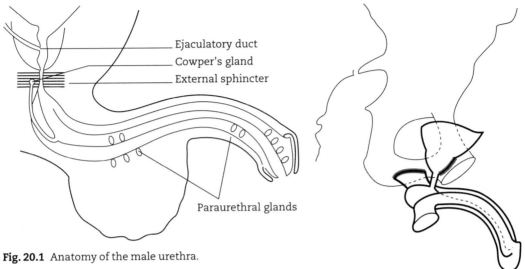

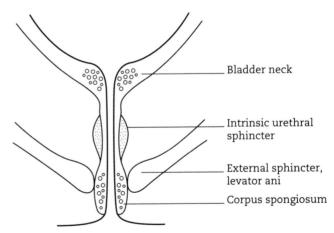

Fig. 20.1 Anatomy of the male urethra.

Fig. 20.2 The fixed attachments of the corpora cavernosa to the ischiopubic rami below and the prostate to the symphysis pubis above: the membranous urethra is the weak link.

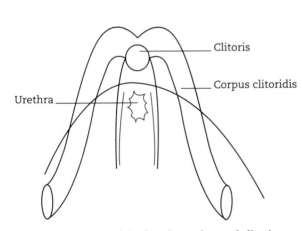

Fig. 20.3 Anatomy of the female urethra and clitoris.

Fig. 20.4 Structure of the female urethra.

CONGENITAL DISORDERS OF THE URETHRA

Errors in the genital folds

HYPOSPADIAS

As the genital folds roll in to form the male urethra and corpus spongiosum they may fail to fuse together, resulting in a urethra opening on the underside of the penis—hypospadias. There are different degrees of hypospadias according to how far down the urethra the defect extends (Fig. 20.5).

Glandular hypospadias (Fig. 20.6). Here the urethra opens on the underside of the glans, but there is no other deformity. It causes no trouble in later life, and it is very questionable whether anything needs to be done about it at all. It can be corrected by an operation, but it is doubtful whether this is justified merely on the basis of some fancied cosmetic advantage.

Penile hypospadias. Here the urethra opens about half-way along the penis. Correction is necessary, and the important thing is to refer the baby to a paediatric urological centre where these operations are done often enough to give the team

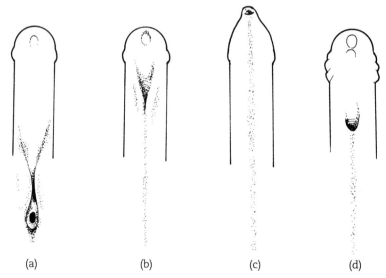

(a)   (b)   (c)   (d)

Fig. 20.5 Incomplete inrolling of the genital folds results in different degrees of hypospadias.

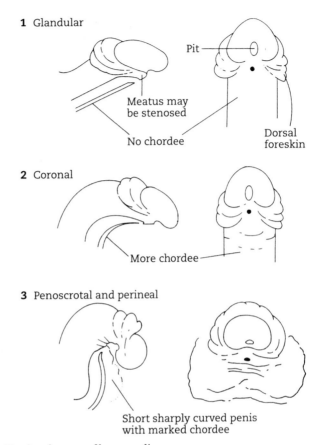

1 Glandular

Pit

Meatus may
be stenosed

No chordee

Dorsal
foreskin

2 Coronal

More chordee

3 Penoscrotal and perineal

Short sharply curved penis
with marked chordee

Fig. 20.6 Varying degrees of hypospadias.

experience. As so often in paediatric urology, this is not a job for the occasional amateur who would like to have a try. In specialized centres a one-stage operation is often successful.

Complete hypospadias. Correction of this deformity is difficult and referral to an expert, who can usually correct the deformity in one stage, is even more necessary.

DUPLEX URETHRA

Wrinkling of the genital folds as they roll in may give rise to a double urethra: it is seldom complete, and the two channels often communicate with the result that the lower one balloons out and obstructs urination (Fig. 20.8).

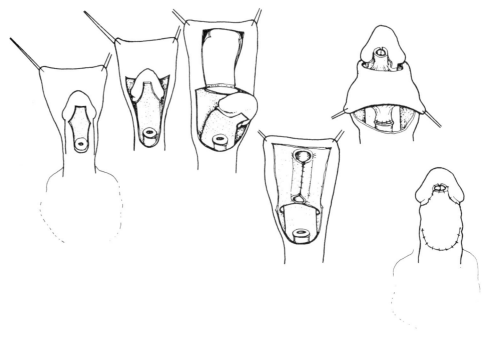

Fig. 20.7 One-stage operation for hypospadias.

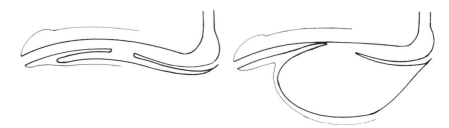

Fig. 20.8 Duplication of the urethra—anterior urethral valve.

Errors in the development of the cloacal membrane

These are dealt with under exstrophy and epispadias, see p. 149.

Congenital posterior urethral valves

The embryological explanation of this anomaly remains a mystery. There is a thin tough membrane just below the verumontanum, with a hole in it like a parachute (Fig. 20.9). It causes obstruction. The bladder goes through all the phases of

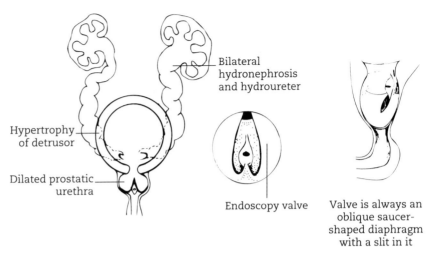

Bilateral
hydronephrosis
and hydroureter

Hypertrophy
of detrusor

Dilated prostatic
urethra

Endoscopy valve

Valve is always an
oblique saucer-
shaped diaphragm
with a slit in it

Fig. 20.9 Congenital posterior urethral valves.

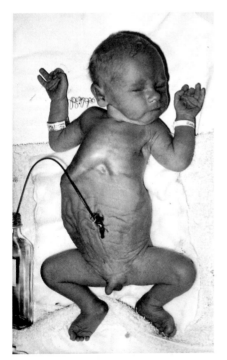

Fig. 20.10 Prune belly syndrome.
Courtesy of Mr J.H. Johnston.

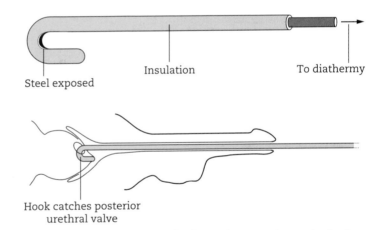

Insulation

To diathermy

Steel exposed

Hook catches posterior
urethral valve

Fig. 20.11 Insulated diathermy hook for destroying posterior urethral valve.

obstruction (see p. 183) responding with hypertrophy, trabeculation, and so on, followed by failure. The condition is often detected in the fetus by ultrasound scanning, and a grommet may be inserted between the distended bladder and the amniotic cavity to relieve the pressure.

Spontaneous cure has been recorded *in utero* when serial ultrasound scans suddenly show the huge bladder to have disappeared.

Prune-belly syndrome

The distended bladder of the fetus squeezes the abdominal wall and prevents ingrowth of muscle from either side. The testicles cannot descend. By the time the baby boy is born the valve is often intact, but sometimes it has ruptured, leaving the prune-belly without an explanation (Fig. 20.10).

Treatment
Once the child has been delivered, nothing is easier than to destroy the little membrane with a hook equipped with diathermy (Fig. 20.11).

TRAUMA

Iatrogenic trauma

Instrumental injury to the urethra is very common. A clean cut will heal with an inconspicuous scar, and no stricture. When the injury is caused by pressure of a catheter leading to ischaemic necrosis—essentially a bedsore—healing leads to a stricture, typically found near the meatus, at the penoscrotal junction, or at the external sphincter (Fig. 20.12).

There is one important variation on this theme. After open heart or aortic surgery multiple strictures occur along the length of the urethra. At first these were thought to be caused by some toxic chemical in latex catheters. Later the same kind of stricture, though less common, was seen with other types of catheter, and it is now thought that the strictures are due to a combination of ischaemia (while the circulation is suspended) and pressure of the catheter, perhaps made worse by chemicals in the material of the catheter itself (Fig. 20.13).

Perineal injury

In past times many a Jack Tar would fall from the rigging of a sailing ship astride a spar, or a Johnny Head-in-Air would trip over a man-hole cover in the street. Today the injury occurs in sport and industry. The blunt force compresses the bulbar urethra up against the inferior edge of the symphysis and tears the corpus spongiosum and urethra (Fig. 20.14). Because the corpus spongiosum is firmly attached to the corpora cavernosa its ends do not retract (Fig. 20.15). Urine and blood escape into the scrotum, in a space limited by the fasciae of Scarpa and Colles, where concentrated or infected urine may cause necrosis of the fat and overlying skin (Fig. 20.16). In neglected cases the entire skin of the scrotum and penis sloughs away, leaving only the testes preserved by the blood supply of the spermatic cord.

MANAGEMENT
The priority is to prevent urine escaping into the scrotum, so a suprapubic tube is

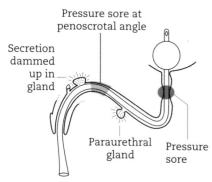

Fig. 20.12 Dangers of a snugly fitting catheter.

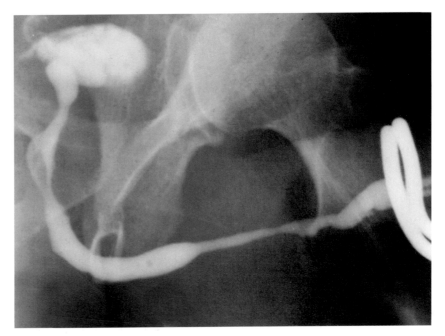

Fig. 20.13 Long urethral stricture following cardiac surgery.

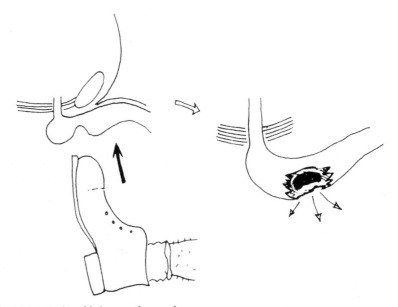

Fig. 20.14 Perineal injury to the urethra.

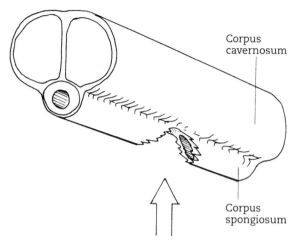

Corpus
cavernosum

Corpus
spongiosum

Fig. 20.15 The attachments to the corpora cavernosa
prevent the ends of the injured urethra from retracting.

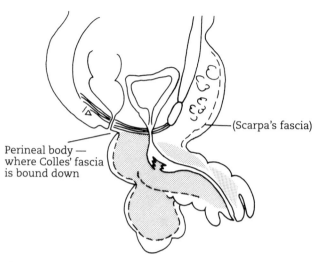

Perineal body —
where Colles' fascia
is bound down

(Scarpa's fascia)

Fig. 20.16 Urine and blood escape into the scrotum and
perineum.

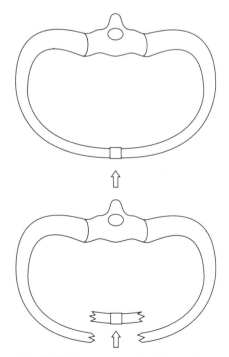

Fig. 20.17 Anteroposterior injury: the
pelvic ring gives way at its thinnest part.

put in the bladder as an emergency. If there is a collection of urine and blood, it
must be drained, but no attempt is made to repair the urethra.

About 10 days later the urethra is examined with the flexible cystoscope: in
nearly every case it will be found to have healed completely. Occasionally the scar
shrinks and causes a stricture, but it is always short and easy to treat.

Fractured pelvis with rupture of the membranous urethra

The membranous urethra is very thin and connects two fixed points, the prostate
above, which is firmly attached to the symphysis, and the bulbar urethra below,
which is bound to the corpus cavernosum on either side which is fixed to the
ischiopubic ramus. If a fracture separates these two fixed points the membranous
urethra is first stretched, and then torn across. There are three types of injury: (i)
minimal displacement of the pelvis; (ii) gross displacement of the pelvis; and (iii)
combined urethral and rectal injuries, e.g. gun-shot wounds.

MINIMAL DISPLACEMENT OF THE PELVIS

When the pelvic ring is compressed from front to back, e.g. by a car backing into a
man leaning over a wall, it gives way where it is thinnest—at the pubic and ischial
rami on either side of the symphysis (Fig. 20.17). The symphysis carries the
prostate back with it while the bulbar urethra remains attached to the ischiopubic

rami. The membranous urethra is first stretched, and may be torn completely or incompletely. The car backs off and the pelvic ring springs back to its original position, but the symphysis is always displaced a little posteriorly. If the lumen of the urethra is intact it will now have an S-shaped bend. If torn completely, the prostatic urethra will come to lie behind the bulb (Fig. 20.18).

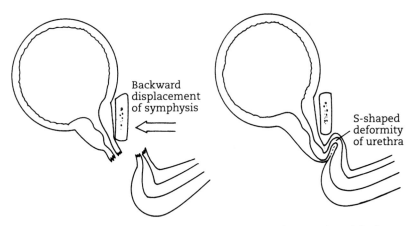

Backward displacement of symphysis

S-shaped deformity of urethra

Fig. 20.18 The displaced segment of pelvic ring returns almost to its original position but the prostatic end now lies posterior to the bulbar end of the ruptured urethra.

Management

In the accident and emergency department X-rays show the typical fracture. Blood escaping from the urethra shows that there has been some damage. About 20 ml of soluble contrast medium is injected into the urethra: extravasation confirms that the urethra has been damaged. At this stage, do not try to pass a catheter: put in a suprapubic tube.

The next step depends on the general state of the patient. Usually there are other more important injuries to be taken care of and it takes several days for the patient to recover sufficiently for the urethral injury to be dealt with. A flexible cystoscope is passed. In an incomplete injury the way can be seen into the bladder and nothing more need be done at this stage. About 2 weeks later the cystoscopy is repeated and at worst may show the S-shaped bend whose thin septa can easily be incised (Fig. 20.19).

If the urethra has been completely torn and the flexible cystoscope does not show any way into the bladder, the bulbar urethra is exposed through a perineal incision, the haematoma is evacuated, and the separated ends are anastomosed together over a silicone catheter (Fig. 20.20). The sooner this can be done the easier it is, but the timing of this operation is nearly always determined by the patient's other injuries.

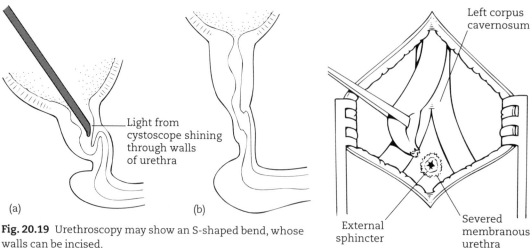

(a)   (b)

Fig. 20.19 Urethroscopy may show an S-shaped bend, whose walls can be incised.

Fig. 20.20 End-to-end anastomosis of the ruptured urethra through a perineal approach.

GROSS DISPLACEMENT OF THE PELVIS

Here the anatomy of the injury is different. The patient has usually been driving a car with an outstretched lower limb, and the force of the impact is transmitted along the limb, forcing the head of the femur through the acetabulum, and dislocating one half of the pelvis upwards, fracturing the pubic and ischial rami and dislocating the sacro-iliac joint (Fig. 20.21). The half pelvis carries up the bladder and prostate. If the bulbar urethra rides up as well, then the urethra escapes damage, but more often the bulbar urethra remains attached to the opposite half of the pelvis and the membranous urethra is torn across. The gap between the severed ends of the urethra is now much wider, and is equal to the distance between the dislocated halves of the pelvis.

Management

In this type of injury the two halves of the pelvis do not spring back together: on the contrary, reduction can be very difficult. There is always tremendous internal haemorrhage from torn pelvic vessels as well as other major injuries, e.g. to the head, liver and chest. For the first 48 h the priority is resuscitation and saving life, but one of the best ways to limit the internal bleeding is to reduce the dislocated pelvis, and maintain the correct position with an external fixator (Fig. 20.22).

From the urologist's point of view, a urethrogram performed (as above) in the accident and emergency department will show whether or not the urethra is damaged. If there is no extravasation, it is safe to pass a urethral catheter. But if there is extravasation, or if there is any doubt, it is better to put in a suprapubic

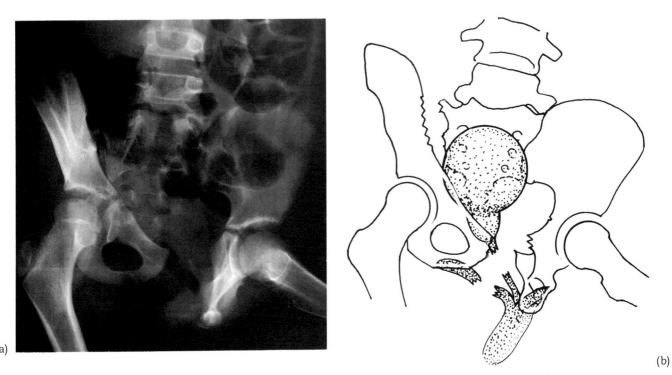

(a)

(b)

Fig. 20.21 Fracture of pelvis wth gross displacement of one half-pelvis.

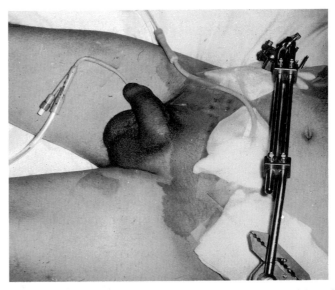

Fig. 20.22 External fixation after reduction of a displaced fracture of the pelvis.

tube. This can be difficult in the presence of the pelvic haematoma, but can be greatly helped by using ultrasound to locate the bladder and make sure the suprapubic tube is in the right position.

Correct reduction of the dislocated pelvis will bring the separated ends of the urethra nearly together. When the general condition of the patient permits, a combination of cystogram and urethrogram (an up-and-down-a-gram) shows where the separated ends of the urethra are lying and an operation is performed to anastomose them together. The timing of this operation is determined by the general condition of the patient, and it is rarely possible for several weeks.

The bulbar urethra is mobilized through a perineal incision, and the prostatic urethra exposed through a retropubic incision. In practice the prostate may have to be mobilized so that the torn ends can be brought together without tension (Fig. 20.23).

Unreduced dislocation
Sometimes it is impossible to effect an accurate reduction of the dislocated half pelvis, and by the time the patient is ready to undergo any urological reconstruction, the pelvis is fixed and the severed ends of the urethra are separated by a long gap. To reconstruct this is exceedingly difficult. Essentially part of the malunited callus has to be removed to allow the mobilized bulbar urethra to be brought up to the lower end of the prostate. There are a number of different methods for doing this, which indicates that none of them is always successful (Fig. 20.24).

COMBINED URETHRAL AND RECTAL INJURIES: GUN-SHOT WOUNDS
These are very rare and very dangerous. The cause is usually a rolling-crushing

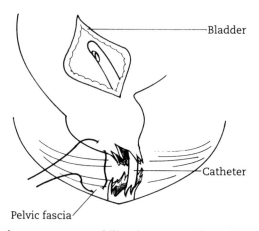

Fig. 20.23 It may be necessary to mobilize the prostate through a retropubic approach.

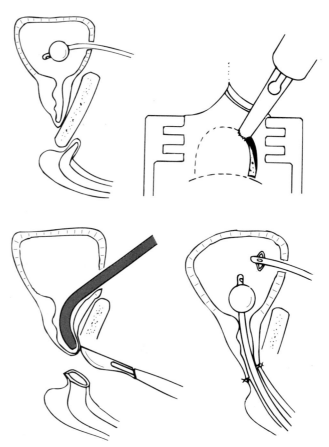

Fig. 20.24 Unreduced displaced fracture of pelvis: end to end anastomosis after removing a window of symphysis.

injury or a gunshot wound (Fig. 20.25). If the rectum is torn, it is essential that faeces are diverted as soon as possible or clostridial infection is likely to lead to gas gangrene. A colostomy is performed as soon as possible, and the distal colon and rectum thoroughly washed out. No attempt is made to perform a primary suture. A careful debridement of the wound is performed, bleeding controlled, and a suprapubic tube inserted. The wound is packed. Plans can then be made for secondary suture and delayed reconstruction.

Complications of urethral injuries

1   *Stricture.* Stricture is a common result of any type of urethral injury.
2   *Impotence.* Impotence can occur after pelvic fractures without urethral injury,

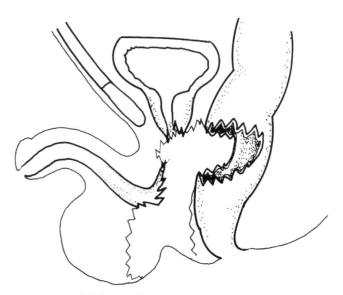

Fig. 20.25 Massive crush injury with laceration of rectum.

and is caused by damage to the neurovascular bundle of the penis or the pelvic autonomic nerves by the fracture and dislocation of the pelvic bones.

3   *Impaired ejaculation.* Damage to the sympathetic nerves may cause paralysis of the bladder neck and seminal vesicles resulting in retrograde or dry ejaculation.

4   *Incontinence.* If the bladder neck has been denervated or destroyed and if the supramembranous intramural sphincter is damaged by the injury, or the attempts to realign the urethra fail, then the patient may be incontinent.

INFLAMMATION OF THE URETHRA

Gonorrhoea has been with mankind from time immemorial. Pharoahs took catheters with them to the after-life, and Socrates made jokes about it. Infection with *Neisseria gonorrhoeae* causes acute inflammation in the periurethral glands. There is a profuse discharge of yellow pus in which a Gram stain will show the typical Gram-negative intracellular diplococci. The patient suffers painful urination, and the oedema and inflammation may cause the penis to bend when erect—*chaudepisse cordée*. Eventually the inflammation subsides, but if not treated promptly with antibiotics, leads to scarring in the periurethral tissues which contracts and causes a stricture (Fig. 20.26).

There are other bacterial causes of urethritis, notably *Chlamydia trachomatis*, in which the organism is more difficult to identify, but which can progress to a stricture.

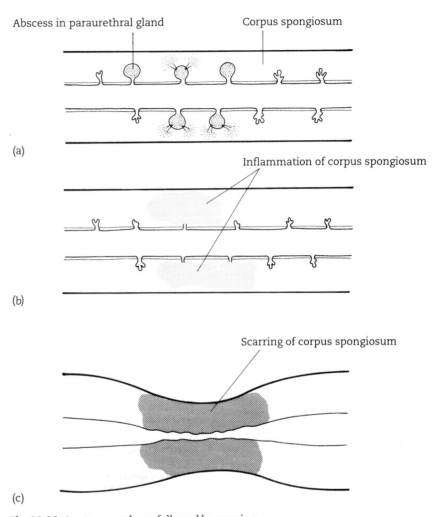

Fig. 20.26 Acute gonorrhoea followed by scarring.

CLINICAL FEATURES OF A STRICTURE

The symptoms of a urethral stricture are those of outflow obstruction, inter-changeable with those where the obstruction is caused by an enlarged prostate (see p. 183).

PHYSICAL SIGNS

There are usually no physical signs, but in long-standing strictures palpation of the urethra will reveal thickening and induration in the corpus spongiosum.

COMPLICATIONS OF A STRICTURE

▮ *Urinary infection.* Infected urine upstream of the urethra, whatever the cause,

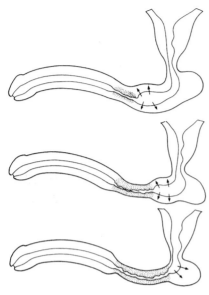

Fig. 20.27 Progression of a stricture.

may be forced into the para-urethral ducts proximal to the stricture and cause further urethritis, and a progression of the stricture along the urethra (Fig. 20.27). Similar intravasation of infected urine may cause prostatitis (see p. 193).

2 *Para-urethral abscess.* An infected para-urethral gland may suppurate, and pus may point in the scrotum, and after it has been incised or has discharged, urine may leak through a fistula. When these are multiple the result is a watering-can perineum. Stones may form in these fistulae (Fig. 20.28).

3 *Sterility.* Even though urine may flow, the thicker semen may be obstructed by the stricture and lead to sterility.

4 *Cancer.* In strictures that have been present for many years, especially when complicated by fistulae, squamous cell cancer may arise.

INVESTIGATION

A flow rate will document the progress of a stricture, but may give a false reassurance that all is well since flow is proportional to the square of the diameter of the urethra.

Urethrography using a water-soluble contrast medium shows the stricture (Fig. 20.29), but not the fibrous changes in the corpus spongiosum, which are better imaged with ultrasound scan (Fig. 20.30). The flexible cystoscope is an easy way to examine the stricture directly.

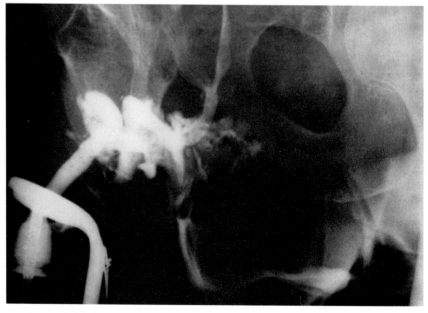

Fig. 20.28 Multiple fistulae after a stricture—watering-can perineum.

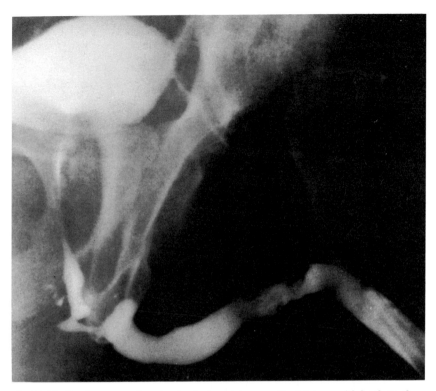

Fig. 20.29 Urethrogram showing typical post-traumatic stricture with backward displacement of upper prostatic part.

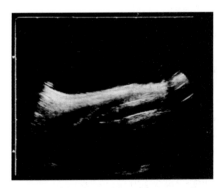

Fig. 20.30 Ultrasound image of urethra showing periurethral fibrosis. Courtesy of Dr W. Hately.

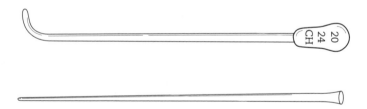

Fig. 20.31 Urethral sound and bougie.

TREATMENT

Regular intermittent dilatation. This is the traditional method of managing a stricture. Ancient instruments were adapted from wax tapers, and the best wax came from the Algerian port of Bujiyah, so flexible dilators are still called bougies even though they are made of plastic, not wax. Curved polished steel dilators are usually called sounds because they resemble the ancient instrument used, before the days of X-rays, to 'sound' for stone in the bladder (Fig. 20.31).

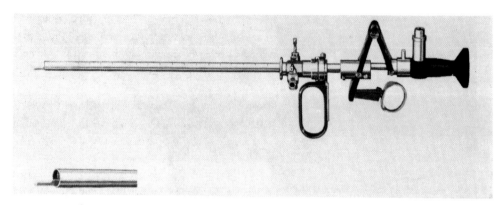

Fig. 20.32 Sachse optical urethrotome. Courtesy of Messrs Rimmer Bros, UK Agents for Karl Storz.

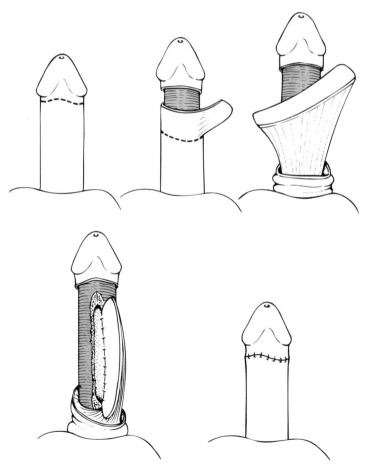

Fig. 20.33 Pedicled skin graft urethroplasty.

Whether flexible or rigid, dilators come in sets of gradually increasing size. They are used to stretch the stricture. Today, patients are given a self-lubricating catheter which they pass on themselves to keep the stricture dilated just as they used to do in ancient Greece.

Internal urethrotomy. When a stricture is too tight to allow a dilator to be passed, the scar tissue is incised under vision with the Sachse optical urethrotome (Fig. 20.32). Urethrotomy is then followed up by regular self-catheterization.

Urethroplasty. To prevent scar tissue from contracting after burns in the skin, plastic surgeons apply a skin graft, and there are many ways of adapting this principle to the urethra. The graft can be made of split skin or whole thickness skin and used as a free graft or on a pedicle of dartos (Fig. 20.33). There are many variations of this principle and the fact that there are so many is sufficient evidence that none of them is completely successful. Urethroplasty is only used when urethrotomy and regular dilatation fail to keep the stricture well controlled.

FURTHER READING

Dineen MD, Duffy PG (1996) Posterior urethral valves. *Br J Urol* **78**: 275.

Halliday P, Doumas K, Prescott S (1996) An audit of urethral stricture management in Lothian. *Br J Urol* **77**: (suppl. p33) 127.

Koraitim MM, Marzouk ME, Atta MA, Orabi SS (1996) Risk factors and mechanism of urethral injury in pelvic fractures. *Br J Urol* **77**: 876.

Mundy AR (1996) Urethroplasty for posterior urethral strictures. *Br J Urol* **78**: 243.

Parkhouse HF, Barratt TM, Dillon MJ *et al.* (1988) Long-term outcome of boys with posterior urethral valves. *Br J Urol* **62**: 59.

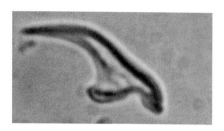

The Penis

SURGICAL ANATOMY

The penis is made of the two corpora cavernosa and the corpus spongiosum surrounding the urethra which expands to form the glans penis (Fig. 21.1). All three are surrounded by the tough rubbery Buck's fascia. When they fill with blood there is an erection. The spongy spaces of the corpora are made of compartments lined with smooth muscle: those of the two corpora cavernosa intercommunicate freely, but not with the corpus spongiosum and glans.

The glans penis is developed from the genital tubercle, into which a tunnel is

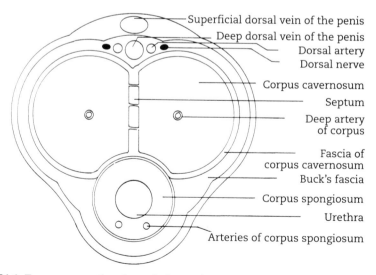

Fig. 21.1 Transverse section through the penis.

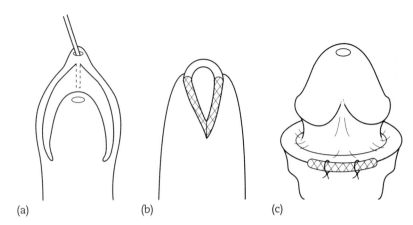

(a)   (b)   (c)

Fig. 21.2 Preputioplasty.

formed during the last stage of the embryological development of the penis. Sometimes this tunnel is imperfect, leading to glandular hypospadias (see p. 218).

A hood of skin then grows over the glans to form the prepuce, and in the later months of fetal life, this hood becomes adherent to the glans, and this congenital adherence only breaks down spontaneously during the first few years of childhood, and almost never causes any trouble.

CIRCUMCISION

The ancient religious rite of circumcision is of great anthropological interest, but is not indicated on any surgical grounds, and is followed by many complications.* True phimosis, i.e. where there is obstruction to the escape of urine from the preputial space, is very rare, and easily dealt with by a small incision in the narrow meatus—preputioplasty (Fig. 21.2).

Balanitis, recurrent inflammation behind a prepuce that cannot be retracted after the age of 5 or 6, can be dealt with by circumcision or preputioplasty, but can usually be avoided by gentle retraction of the prepuce in the bath.

Blood supply

ARTERIES

The penis receives blood from three terminal branches of the internal pudendal

---

* The arguments for and against neonatal circumcision have been raging for many centuries, with passion inversely proportional to reason:
Editorial (1979) The case against neonatal circumcision. *Br Med J* **1**: 1163.
Gordon A, Collin J (1993) Save the normal foreskin. *Br Med J* **306**: 1.
Duckett JW (1995) A temperate approach to neonatal circumcision. *Urology* **46**: 771.
Dresner ML (1995) Circumcision in infancy. *Urology* **46**: 769.

artery (Fig. 21.3) on each side: the deep arteries of the corpora, the dorsal arteries, and the bulbourethral arteries.

VEINS

There are three groups of veins (Fig. 21.4).

1   The deep dorsal veins drain the corpora cavernosa and lead under the symphysis pubis into the large veins which surround the prostate and bladder.

2   The superficial veins, under the skin, mostly drain into the saphenous veins.

3   The intermediate veins, deep to Buck's fascia, drain blood from the glans penis into both deep and superficial systems.

NERVES

Sensation. Sensation from the penis is carried in the dorsal nerves which run beside each dorsal artery to join the pudendal nerve (S2, S3).

Motor nerves. The cavernous nerves carry parasympathetic fibres in two discrete bundles on either side of the prostate, surrounding the arteries. Care is taken to preserve them in the operation of radical nerve-sparing prostatectomy (see p. 211).

PHYSIOLOGY OF ERECTION

Flaccid state

The flaccid penis has a relatively low blood flow through its spongy tissues.

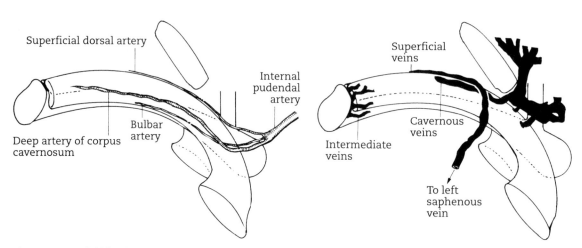

Fig. 21.3 Arterial blood supply to the penis.

Fig. 21.4 Venous drainage of the penis.

Tumescence

Parasympathetic stimulation, mediated by neurotransmitter substances (whose action is imitated by papaverine, phentolamine and prostaglandin E), causes the small branches of the deep arteries of the corpora cavernosa to dilate and fill the spaces of the spongy tissue with blood, while their smooth muscle walls relax. The pressure inside the corpus cavernosum rises to about 40 mmHg (Fig. 21.5).

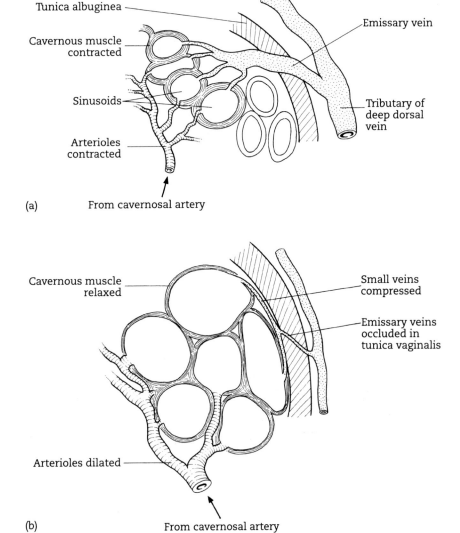

Fig. 21.5 Mechanism of erection. (a) Flaccid; (b) erect.

Rigidity

During the third phase of erection further parasympathetic stimulation occludes the veins leading out of the corpora cavernosa and spongiosum trapping blood inside them. The pressure rises inside the corpora to over 150 mmHg.

EJACULATION

There are five steps in ejaculation (Fig. 21.6). The first four are under autonomic control: the fifth is mediated by somatic motor components in the pudendal nerve.

1   The seminal vesicles pump themselves up.

2   The bladder neck contracts.

3   The vas deferens undergoes peristalsis, ejecting 0.5 ml of fluid containing its store of sperms.

4   The seminal vesicles expel their contents.

5   The bulbospongiosus muscles contract repeatedly to squeeze the semen out from the bulbar urethra.

ERECTILE IMPOTENCE

Unrealistic expectations

Some men consult the doctor because they feel their performance is below par, e.g. if they cannot ejaculate more than three times per night. Age brings a normal diminution in sexual activity.

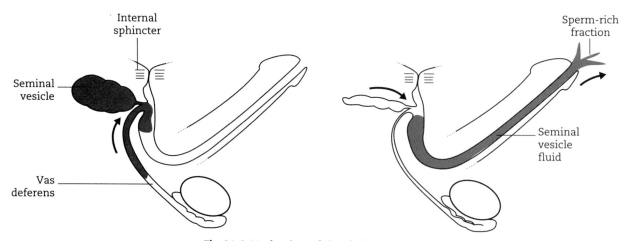

Fig. 21.6 Mechanism of ejaculation.

Wrong partner

Some patients can ejaculate perfectly well in their dreams or on masturbation and with one partner but not another. This is a psychological minefield and expert counselling is essential.

No desire

Many patients wake with an erection in the morning, but with no desire for intercourse. Sometimes this is a feature of overwork: frustration, alcohol and divorce are common features of the syndrome. A holiday may cure the condition, but expert counselling may be needed.

No erection at all

There are a number of organic causes for malfunction of the physiology of erection, e.g. arterial obstruction (diabetes and arteriosclerosis); parasympathetic disorders (diabetes, Shy–Drager syndrome); pelvic trauma involving the autonomic nerves, or surgery in the pelvis; or medication especially with antidepressant drugs.

Investigation

The investigation of organic impotence should proceed in logical steps. Diabetes is easily excluded. Obstruction to the blood supply of the penis can be tested by Doppler studies of the penile blood flow or by a test injection into the corpus cavernosum of one of the substances that mimics parasympathetic stimulation, e.g. papaverine or prostaglandin E. Nocturnal tumescence, which accompanies dreaming in the phase of sleep marked by rapid eye movements, can be monitored by means of paper strips (Fig. 21.7) or an electronic device (Fig. 21.8). Failure of the occlusion of the penile veins during the third, rigid phase of erection—venous leakage—can be diagnosed by injecting contrast into the corpora cavernosa while monitoring the pressure, as an artificial erection is produced by prostaglandin injection (Fig. 21.9).

Treatment

1   *Yohimbine* is an alkaloid similar to reserpine, and may in some cases restore erection if given as 5 mg three times per day.

2   *Vacuum devices* are available which suck blood into the penis to produce an artificial tumescence which is then maintained with a rubber band around the base of the penis. Many patients find this satisfactory.

3   *Self-injection.* If a test injection of prostaglandin E produces a successful erection, the patient can be taught to do it himself. It is essential that he knows who to telephone if the erection fails to subside after 3 or 4 h so that the condition can be promptly corrected (see *priapism*, p. 244).

4   *Implanted penile prostheses.* Devices are available which can be inserted into

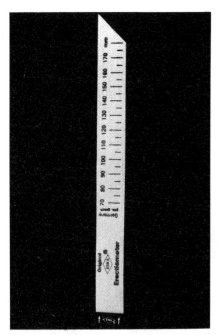

Fig. 21.7 Paper strip to record expansion of penis during sleep.

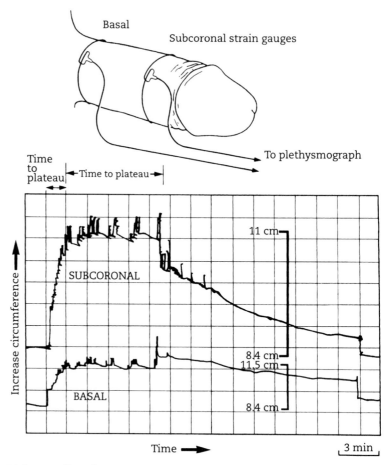

Fig. 21.8 Recording of tumescence and elongation of penis. Courtesy of Mr P. Blacklay.

the corpora cavernosa to stiffen them. Some can be bent and made to straighten out, others are inflated from a concealed reservoir. They are all expensive, and their insertion calls for great care. Being a mechanical foreign body, there is a high risk of infection, erosion and mechanical failure (Fig. 21.10).

5 *Vascular operations* are under trial: in the first type the inferior epigastric artery is anastomosed to the dorsal artery of the penis. In the second the objective is to prevent blood leaking out of the penis when a venous leak has been demonstrated.

EJACULATORY FAILURE

Premature ejaculation
The problem here is a trigger that is too sensitive: it is not physiologically

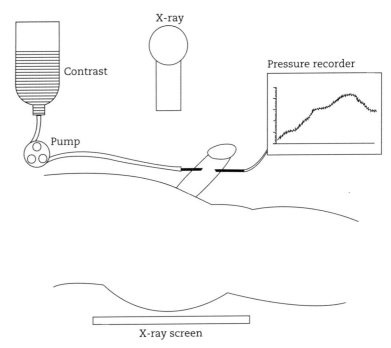

Fig. 21.9 Corpus cavernosography.

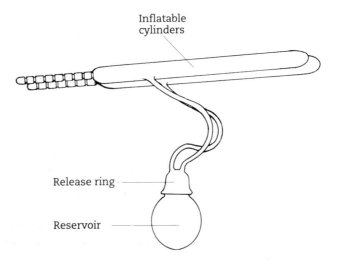

Fig. 21.10 Inflatable penile prosthesis. (Surgitek Uniflate 1000.)

abnormal. Counselling may help, but the most simple remedy is to let the couple have a rest and try again at some convenient later time.

Inhibited ejaculation

Guilt, anxiety, a squeaky bed, fear of discovery—most young lovers and all novelists know how such factors can inhibit lovemaking. A counsellor may help.

No ejaculation

1   The seminal tract may be blocked at the ejaculatory ducts. Ejaculation may be painful. A transrectal ultrasound may show distended seminal vesicles. It may be possible to unblock the ejaculatory ducts by incision or resection of their openings on the verumontanum.

2   A urethral stricture may prevent the escape of semen. The obstruction is cured by treating the stricture (see p. 232).

3   Retrograde ejaculation may be taking place because of previous surgery at the bladder neck, or because the sympathetic innervation of the bladder neck has been destroyed by trauma or surgery in the pelvis, or by medication with an α-blocker. A sympathomimetic drug may cure the problem.

Priapism

In priapism the corpora cavernosa are rigid, but the glans penis is soft. There are two types of priapism:

1   *Low flow priapism*. This may occur after normal intercourse, after medication with α-blocking drugs such as prazosin, and in certain haematological conditions, e.g. sickle cell disease, leukaemia, and in patients undergoing haemodialysis. It is most often seen after self-injection with papaverine or prostaglandin E for impotence.

2   *High flow priapism*. This is rare, and occurs when injury has led to an aneurysm of the deep artery of the corpus cavernosum. A Doppler study will show the high blood flow and measurement of the pO_2 of blood aspirated from the penis will show that it resembles arterial blood.

TREATMENT

In low flow priapism due to leukaemia and dialysis, no treatment is required other than bed rest and analgesia. In sickle cell disease plasmapheresis can be used to rid the blood of misshapen red cells.

In the other more common forms of priapism intracavernosal injection of noradrenaline or aramine is given and usually rapidly reverses the process. If this fails, a hole is made between the flaccid glans penis or corpus spongiosum and the rigid corpora cavernosa either with a biopsy needle (Fig. 21.11) or by surgical anastomosis. The treatment is a matter of urgency because delay may be followed

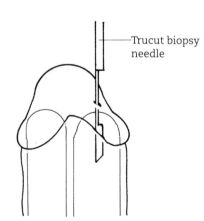

Trucut biopsy needle

Fig. 21.11 Hole made between glans penis and corpus cavernosum with biopsy needle.

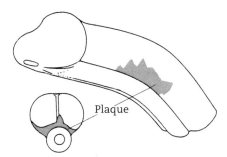

Fig. 21.12 Peyronie's disease.

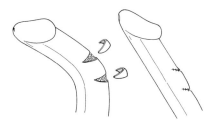

Fig. 21.13 Correction of the curvature in Peyronie's disease.

by irreversible changes in the lining of the sinuses of the spongy tissue of the corpora leading to permanent erectile impotence.

PEYRONIE'S DISEASE

Plaques of fibrous tissue develop in Buck's fascia or the septum between the corpora cavernosa (Fig. 21.12). During an erection the part affected by fibrosis does not fill so the penis bends over. The cause is not known. It may occur in association with similar lumps of fibrous tissue in the palms of the hands (Dupuytren's contracture), nodules in the ears and retroperitoneal fibrosis.

The treatment of Peyronie's disease offers rich pickings to the quack: everything from acupuncture to radiotherapy has been used. The latest in a long line of medications is tamoxifen, which is said to be promising. Whatever treatment is given, in many cases the discomfort ceases and the deformity reduces spontaneously. Large lumps of fibrous tissue disappear. Frequently all that the patient needs is reassurance.

When the condition is particularly painful, or the angulation of the penis prevents intercourse, the penis can be straightened by taking a series of tucks in the tunica on the side opposite to the plaque (Fig. 21.13).

INFLAMMATION OF THE PENIS

ACUTE BALANITIS

Acute balanitis occurs in men who cannot retract the foreskin to keep the preputial space and glans penis clean. It can be due to a specific infection, e.g. *Haemophilus ducreyii*, which causes chancroid, and *Candida albicans*, which occurs particularly commonly in diabetic men. Recurrent acute balanitis is one indication for therapeutic circumcision (see below).

Ulceration on the glans penis may be due to primary infection with syphilis, in which case the spirochaetes of *Treponema pallidum* can be identified in the serum which is expressed from the ulcer. Its diagnosis and treatment is a matter for the appropriate experts to whom the patient should be referred.

CANCER OF THE PENIS

AETIOLOGY

Cancer of the penis occurs in uncircumcised men who are usually old and unwashed and whose foreskin has never been pulled back to keep the glans clean.

There has been endless debate over the issue of preventing cancer of the penis by routine neonatal circumcision. Childhood circumcision certainly does prevent cancer of the penis, but has its own mortality and morbidity, and it has been calculated that slightly more deaths would occur if all boys were to be circumcised than would occur from cancer of the penis, at least in the West. Soap and water appear to be just as effective in preventing penile cancer.

Smoking and previous recurrent balanitis are predisposing factors, as are four well-recognized conditions:

1 *Erythroplasia of Queyrat.* This is a form of carcinoma *in situ* of the skin of the glans. It resembles balanitis, and is diagnosed by means of a biopsy. It can be cured with local coagulation with a CO_2 laser, or 5-fluorouracil cream. If it is neglected it progresses to overt cancer (Fig. 21.14).

2 *Balanitis xerotica obliterans.* This is a skin condition, identical with lichen sclerosus et obliterans. It is common, and usually benign, but may procede to cancer and should always be followed up. There is a whitish alteration in the skin of the prepuce causing it to become stiff, tight and difficult to retract. When the condition affects the glans penis it produces a stenosis of the external urinary meatus which may require surgical correction (Fig. 21.15).

3 *Condyloma acuminatum.* This is a benign wart caused by one of the family of papilloma viruses (Fig. 21.16) which responds to local measures such as podophyllin, freezing and diathermy.

4 *Occasionally condyloma acuminatum* is seen in a giant form, the *Buschke–Loewenstein tumour.* At first this contains papilloma virus and seems histologically to be benign, but if not treated radically always progresses to invasive cancer.

PATHOLOGY

Cancer of the penis occurs in three macroscopic forms, an ulcer, a papilliferous

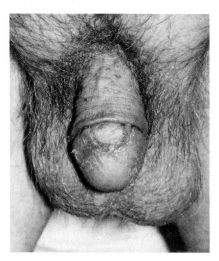

Fig. 21.14 Erythroplasia of Queyrat.

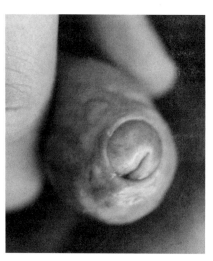

Fig. 21.15 Balanitis xerotica obliterans.

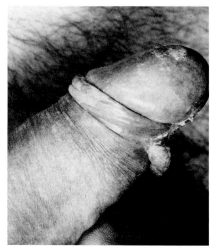

Fig. 21.16 Condyloma acuminatum.

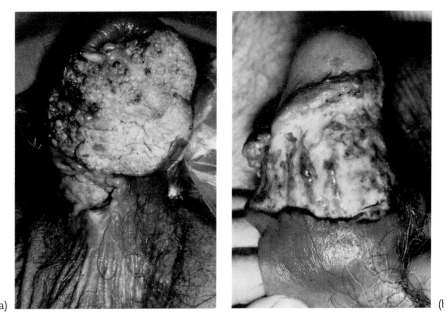

(a)   (l

Fig. 21.17 Papillary and ulcerated types of carcinoma of the penis.

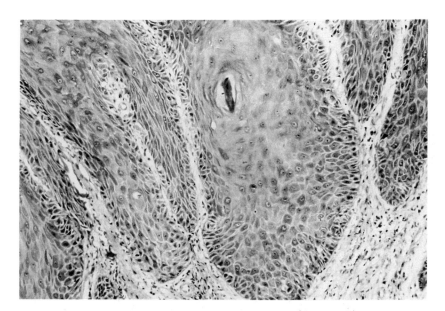

Fig. 21.18 Squamous cell carcinoma of penis. Courtesy of Dr Jo Martin.

cauliflower or a nodule (Fig. 21.17). There is always secondary infection, and many of these cases present late in the course of the disease with a profuse, evil-smelling discharge from beneath an inflamed prepuce.

Grade

These are all squamous cell cancers. There are three histological grades of tumour, G1–G3, according to the frequency of mitoses that are present (Fig. 21.18).

Stage

See Fig. 21.19.

Diagnosis

At first the diagnosis is in doubt, and the first step is a circumcision to uncover the tumour and obtain a biopsy. At this stage there is usually much secondary infection and the inguinal lymph nodes are often enlarged because of inflammation.

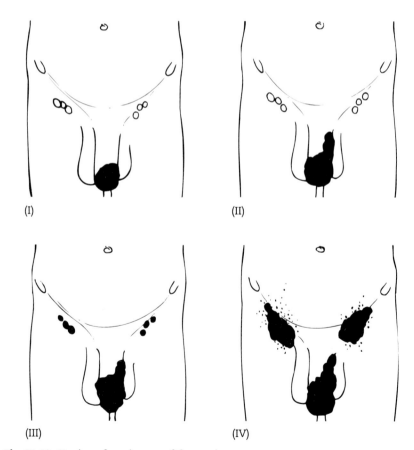

(I)

(II)

(III)

(IV)

Fig. 21.19 Staging of carcinoma of the penis.

Treatment

Stage I
If not entirely removed by circumcision, the choice of treatment is partial amputation (Fig. 21.20) or local radiotherapy. Both can produce 100% cure and after radiotherapy there is a 20% chance of local recurrence that eventually requires partial amputation.

Stage II
Local radiation still offers 100% cure, but 50% will require partial amputation for residual or recurrent disease. Preliminary radiation improves the long-term survival. It is important to know that even after partial amputation patients can still enjoy a normal sex life.

Stage III
If the scrotum is involved wide radical excision offers an excellent chance of cure.

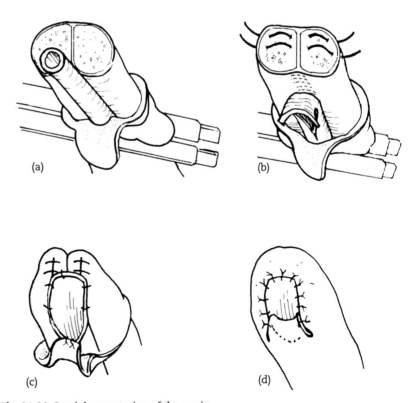

Fig. 21.20 Partial amputation of the penis.

Stage IV
When the inguinal nodes are involved, as may be shown by cytological examination of fluid aspirated from an inguinal node, computed tomography scanning is performed to detect involvement of nodes along the iliac vessels and aorta. Treatment is by a combination of chemotherapy and block dissection of all the nodes that are found to be involved. The major complication of block dissection of the inguinal lymph nodes is distressing oedema of the lower limb, which can only in part be prevented or relieved by supportive stockings.

FURTHER READING

Duckett JW (1995) Circumcision in infancy. *Urology* **46**: 769.

Dunsmuir WD, Kirby RS (1996) Francois de La Peyronie (1678–1747): the man and the disease he described. *Br J Urol* **78**: 613.

Flynn RJ, Williams G (1996) Long-term follow-up of patients with erectile dysfunction commenced on self injection with intracavernosal papaverine with or without phentolamine. *Br J Urol* **78**: 628.

Gairdner D (1949) The fate of the foreskin. *Br Med J* **2**: 1433.

Hellstrom WJG, Bennett AH, Gesundheit N *et al.* (1996) A double-blind, placebo-controlled evaluation of the erectile response to transurethral alprostadil. *Urology* **48**: 851.

Lindegaard JC, Nielsen OS, Lundbeck FA, Mamsen A, Studstrup NH, von der Maase H (1996) A retrospective analysis of 82 cases of cancer of the penis. *Br J Urol* **77**: 883.

Neulander E, Walfisch, S, Kaneti J (1996) Amputation of distal penile glans during neonatal ritual circumcision—a rare complication. *Br J Urol* **77**: 924.

Remondino PC (1891) *History of Circumcision*. Philadelphia, Davis.

Shulman J, Ben-Hur N, Neuman Z (1964) Surgical complications of circumcision. *Am J Dis Child* **107**: 149.

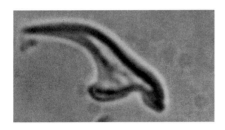

The Testicle

EMBRYOLOGY

The germ cells arise in the yolk sac of the fetus, migrate along the umbilical cord, and bury themselves in the gonadal ridge on the back of the coelom (Fig. 22.1). Later the future testis bulges forwards, and then follows a lump of jelly called the

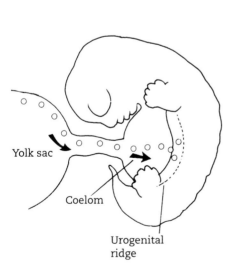

Fig. 22.1 The incredible journey of the germinal cells from the yolk sac to the urogenital ridge.

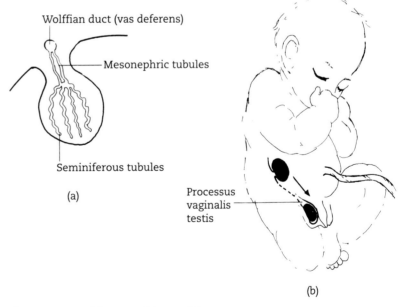

Fig. 22.2 Normal descent of the testicle.

gubernaculum downwards into the scrotum, carrying with it a bag of peritoneum in front and reaching the scrotum shortly before birth (Fig. 22.2).

SURGICAL ANATOMY

The term testicle includes both testis and epididymis. The testis lies in front of the epididymis, slung from the external inguinal ring by the spermatic cord. In front of the testis and nearly surrounding it is the tunica vaginalis, remnant of the peritoneum. It contains only a trace of fluid (Fig. 22.3).

BLOOD SUPPLY

The testicular artery arises from the aorta near the renal arteries and passes in front of the ureter and curls round lateral to the inferior epigastric vessels to enter the inguinal canal. The numerous large veins which drain the testicle form the pampiniform plexus which join together to enter the vena cava on the right and the renal vein on the left (Fig. 22.4).

STRUCTURE

Each testis is made up of sets of tubules arranged in loops, which empty into a sac, the rete testis, which drains through a dozen vasa efferentia into the epididymis (Fig. 22.5). The testicular tubule contains two types of cell — germinal cells and

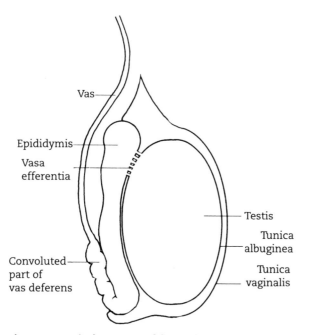

Fig. 22.3 Surgical anatomy of the testicle.

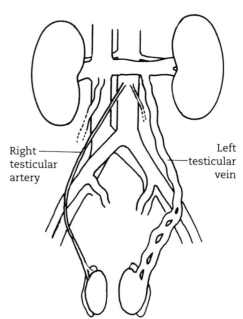

Fig. 22.4 Blood supply of the testicle.

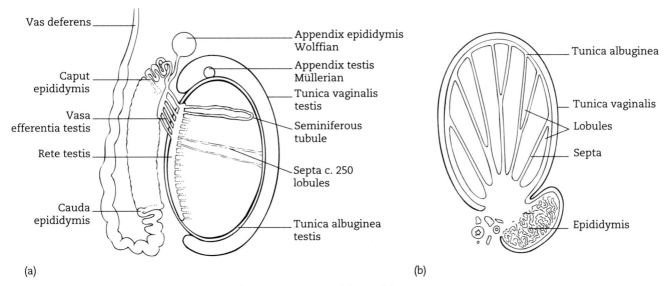

Fig. 22.5 Structure of the testicle.

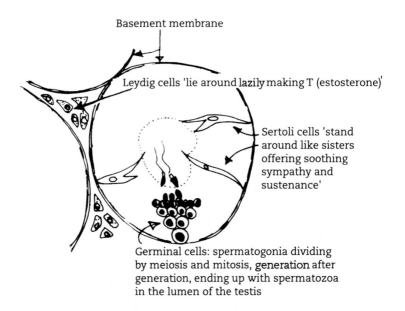

Fig. 22.6 Diagram of testicular tubule.

Sertoli cells. In between them there is a packing of Leydig cells (Fig. 22.6). The germinal cells divide into successive generations of spermatocytes which ultimately develop by mitosis and meiosis into spermatozoa (Fig. 22.7).

The Sertoli cells secrete inhibin which regulates the pituitary supply of luteinizing hormone (Fig. 22.8). The Leydig cells secrete testosterone.

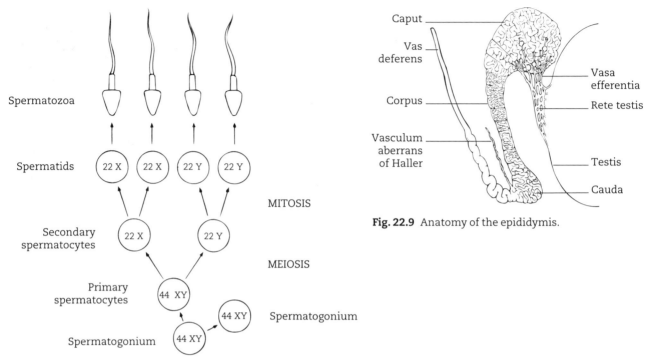

Fig. 22.7 Spermatogenesis.

Fig. 22.9 Anatomy of the epididymis.

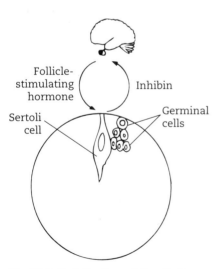

Fig. 22.8 Sertoli cells and the pituitary.

The epididymis is a long coiled tube lying behind the testis, which continues as the vas deferens. It is lined with microcilia similar to those in the bronchioles (Fig. 22.9).

The vas deferens runs along the back of the spermatic cord, curls around the inferior epigastric vessels, crosses in front of the ureter and passes in the cleft between the inner and outer zones of the prostate to join the common ejaculatory duct and open into the prostatic urethra on the verumontanum. The vas deferens has a powerful muscular wall, and is lined with columnar epithelium. It acts as a reservoir for sperms, emptying on ejaculation (Fig. 22.10).

The seminal vesicle lies behind the prostate, just under the bladder. It is a long duct, coiled up so that on cross-section it resembles a honeycomb. Its duct joins the vas deferens to form the common ejaculatory duct (Fig. 22.11).

Congenital anomalies of the testicle

UNDESCENDED TESTICLE

There are two kinds of undescended testicle, those in which the gubernaculum

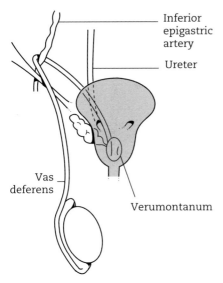

Fig. 22.10 Surgical anatomy of the vas deferens.

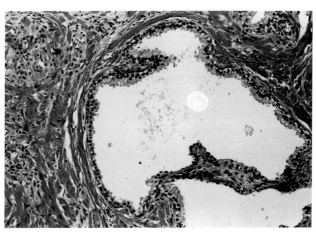

Fig. 22.11 Histology of seminal vesicle. Courtesy of Dr Suhail Baithun.

has gone off course—ectopic—and those in which the descent to the bottom of the scrotum is incomplete—incomplete descent (Fig. 22.12).

Ectopic testicle

Ectopic testicles may be (i) in the abdominal wall near the external inguinal ring—perineal; (ii) penile, near the base of the penis; or (iii) crural, in the thigh (Fig. 22.13).

Incomplete descent

These testicles always move up and down, and are defined according to their range of movement as (i) *abdominal*, usually just inside the internal inguinal ring; (ii) *inguinal*, in the inguinal canal; (iii) *emergent*, when they appear at the external ring; (iv) *high retractile*, when they move up and down but cannot be made to go to the bottom of the scrotum; and (v) *low retractile*, when they descend to the bottom of the scrotum in a warm bath, under general anaesthesia, or with a little gentle persuasion by a doctor with a warm hand.

Difficulty occurs in making the diagnosis of the low retractile testis, which is essentially normal, and will always end up in the scrotum with puberty.

Complications

I   Torsion. There is often a large loose sac of peritoneum in front of an emergent

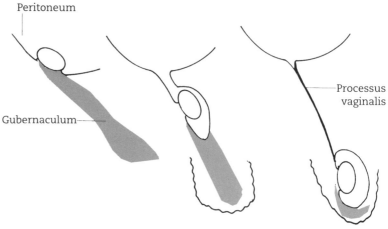

Fig. 22.12 The gubernaculum opens the way for the testicle to follow into the scrotum.

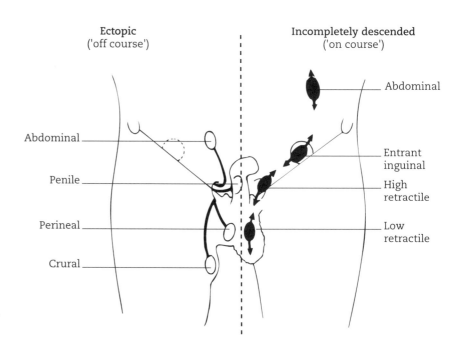

Fig. 22.13 Undescended testicles may be off or on course.

or retractile undescended testicle which makes it prone to torsion (see below) (Fig. 22.14).

2   Infertility. Infertility is common with bilateral undescended testicles, but not with unilateral undescent.

3   Cancer. About one in 10 testicular tumours is associated with maldescent (see p. 266).

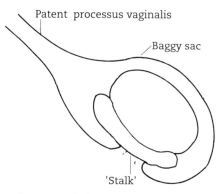

Fig. 22.14 The baggy peritoneal sac associated with incomplete descent favours torsion.

Diagnosis

In most cases the diagnosis is made by inspection and palpation. Difficulty may arise with the low retractile testis: seldom is this difficult for an experienced doctor with warm hands, and a child who is not frightened. When in doubt the child should be examined in a warm bath, and if there is still doubt, given a general anaesthetic to see if the testicle descends to the bottom of the scrotum.

When no testicle can be felt on one side, it is often in the inguinal canal. The testicle is easily found with a computed tomography (CT) scan, even in the abdomen.

Management

Ectopic testes
These never find their way into the scrotum and require orchiopexy.

Incomplete descent
I Abdominal. These are now located by CT scan, if necessary confirmed by laparoscopy. In prepubertal boys an effort should be made to preserve the testis. In the Fowler–Stephens procedure the testicular artery is divided as a first step which may be performed through a laparoscope (Fig. 22.15). Some 6 months later at a second operation the testicle is mobilized and brought down into the scrotum, by which time it will have acquired a new blood supply from the artery to the vas (Fig. 22.16).

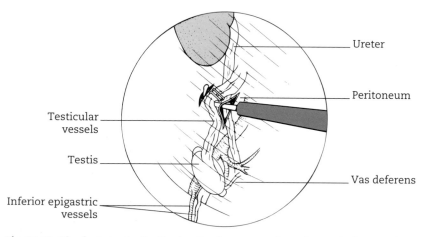

Fig. 22.15 The first step in the Fowler–Stephens procedure: the testicular vessels are clipped laparoscopically.

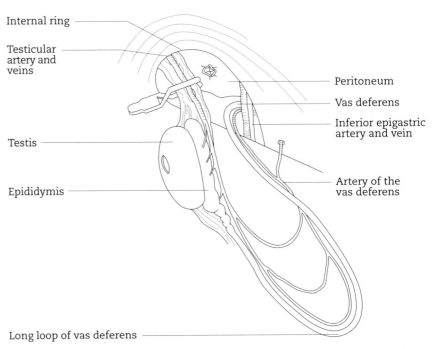

Internal ring

Testicular
artery and
veins

Testis

Epididymis

Peritoneum

Vas deferens

Inferior epigastric
artery and vein

Artery of the
vas deferens

Long loop of vas deferens

Fig. 22.16 Second stage in the Fowler–Stephens procedure: the testicular vessels
are divided and the testicle brought down.

2   Inguinal. Most of these are brought down by the routine operation of
orchiopexy.

Orchiopexy. Through a crease incision over the internal ring, the external oblique
is opened, the testicle is mobilized taking great care not to injure its artery or the
vas deferens. The testicular vessels are followed up behind the peritoneum and
mobilized medially, allowing the testicle to be placed in a sac between the dartos
muscle and skin of the scrotum without tension (Fig. 22.17).

Hormone treatment. Puberty can be brought on early by giving pituitary
gonadotrophins, which accelerate the descent of a low retractile testis but at the
price of premature puberty and stunting of growth from early fusion of epiphyses.
The method is no longer used.

Timing of orchiopexy. Although 90% of testicles are in the scrotum at birth, the
next 9% do not descend until 12 months, after which no more do. Infertility, and
possibly the late development of cancer, is thought to be prevented by orchiopexy
performed before the age of 3, so the window of opportunity is between 2 and 3,

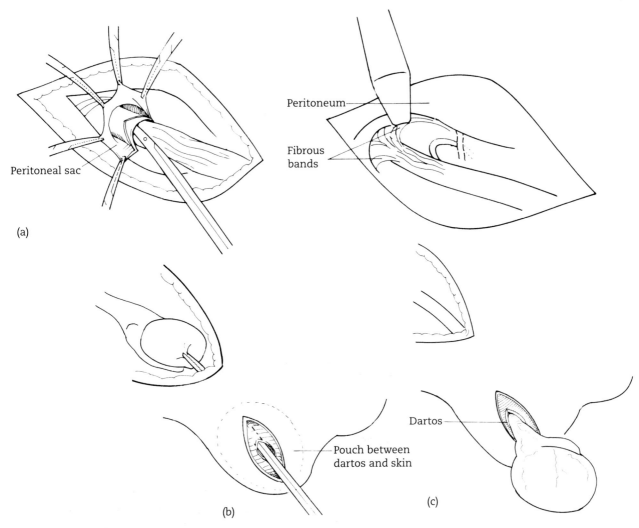

Fig. 22.17 Orchiopexy.

but at this age the technique is difficult. The best results are only obtained in specialized paediatric centres.

After puberty the chance of improving fertility is minimal, and the risk of cancer increases rapidly, but most young men wish to keep both testes.

When an undescended testicle is found in a mature grown man orchiectomy is the procedure that should be advised in view of the risks of malignancy. If the patient is concerned about his cosmetic appearance he may be offered a silicone prosthesis.

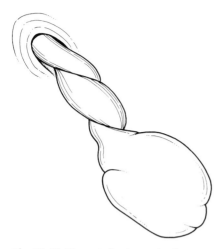

Fig. 22.18 Neonatal extravaginal torsion.

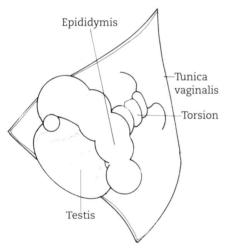

Fig. 22.19 Intravaginal torsion of the testicle.

TORSION

EXTRAVAGINAL

This is seen in newborn boys. The testicle has rotated on the spermatic cord and it is almost never possible to save the testis by untwisting it (Fig. 22.18).

INTRAVAGINAL

The tunica vaginalis may be unusually roomy even with a normally descended testicle, and the testis and epididymis can twist on a stalk like a light-bulb in its socket (Fig. 22.19). Patients often recall attacks of pain that come on and are relieved equally suddenly, and a history of such warning attacks is sufficient reason to explore the testicle and fix it.

Torsion may occur at any age, but is most common around puberty.

Clinical features

There is a sudden onset of pain and swelling in the testicle which may wake the boy. On examination the scrotum is tender, red and swollen, and it is seldom possible to make out testis from epididymis (Fig. 22.20).

The differential diagnosis is from:
1 mumps orchitis, which never attacks boys before puberty;
2 epididymitis, which is always secondary to obvious urinary infection;
3 fat necrosis, which is occasionally seen in infants;
4 cancer, which in older boys and men can present with inflammation;
5 torsion of an appendix testis. This cannot be distinguished from torsion of the testis without exploration.

Investigations

It is important to untwist the testicle before it dies from ischaemia, and no investigation should be allowed to delay surgical exploration. A Doppler or radio-isotope scan may show absence of arterial circulation in the testicle but is justified only if it will not delay matters.

Treatment

The testicle is explored through a transverse scrotal incision. The tunica vaginalis is opened, and the testicle is untwisted. If there is any doubt about the viability of the testis it can be incised to see if it still bleeds. All too often it is necrotic and must be removed.

Because torsion occurs in about 10% of cases on the other side, it is usual to fix the other testicle at the same time.

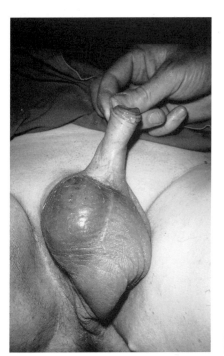

Fig. 22.20 Appearance of torsion of the testicle.

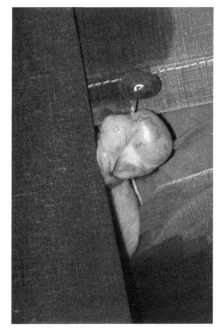

Fig. 22.21 Torsion of an appendix testis.

Torsion of the appendix testis

Tiny cysts are usually present at the upper pole, one on the epididymis (of Wolffian duct origin), the other on the testis (of Müllerian duct origin). Apart from being of interest to embryologists either can twist on its stalk, exactly mimicking torsion of the testicle and equally requiring urgent exploration (Fig. 22.21).

VARICOCELE

The normal pampiniform plexus of veins draining the testicle has been thought to act as a heat-exchanger to keep the testicle cool. A varicocele is a physiological dilatation of these veins (Fig. 22.22). It is widely believed to depress spermatogenesis and lead to atrophy of the testis, and many operations are performed for this reason although every controlled study so far has shown that the operations make no difference. The testicular vessels are approached through a short incision above and parallel to the inguinal ligament, the veins are separated from the testicular artery, ligated and divided. It has become fashionable to do the same thing via a laparoscope.*

HYDROCELE

Fluid accumulates in the cavity of the tunica vaginalis testis as a result of obstruction to the lymphatic drainage of the testicle, in oedema caused by heart failure or as a secondary effusion when there is disease in the testis or epididymis (Fig. 22.23).

NEONATAL

When a hydrocele in a neonate is associated with a hernia, it is operated on almost as an emergency in view of the risk of strangulation. The processus vaginalis is found at the external ring and ligated. There is no need to do anything about the tunica vaginalis testis (Fig. 22.24).

ADULT

In an adult the fear is that the hydrocele may be concealing some mischief in the

---

* Surgical correction of varicocele is very often done for infertility, but on virtually no evidence:

Hargreave TB and WHO Task Force (1996) The World Health Organization varicocele trial. *Br J Urol* 77: 39. (160).

Jarow JP, Coburn M, Sigman M (1996) Incidence of varicoceles in men with primary and secondary infertility. *Urology* 47: 73–6.

Nilsson S, Edvinsson A, Nilsson B (1979) Improvement of semen and pregnancy rate after ligation and division of the internal spermatic vein: fact or fiction? *Br J Urol* 51: 591.

Vermeulen A, Vandeweghe M (1984) Improved fertility after varicocele correction: fact or fiction? *Fertil Steril* 42: 249.

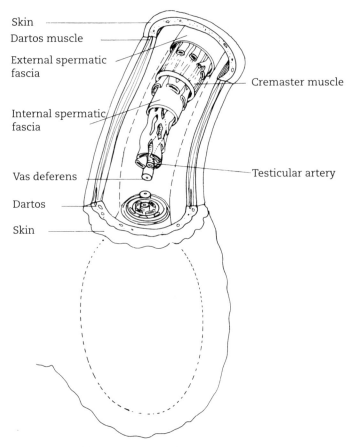

Skin
Dartos muscle
External spermatic
fascia
Cremaster muscle
Internal spermatic
fascia
Vas deferens
Testicular artery
Dartos
Skin

Fig. 22.22 The veins of the spermatic cord.

testis. Ultrasound screening is performed to ensure that the testis is healthy, and if there is any doubt, tumour markers are measured to rule out cancer of the testis (see p. 267).

Few hydroceles need any treatment: a good rule is to offer an operation if the patient's wife or his tailor complain. The options are to aspirate the fluid (Fig. 22.25) or to remove the surplus tunica vaginalis (Fig. 22.26).

CYSTS OF THE EPIDIDYMIS

A few tiny cysts are always present in the upper end of the epididymis, arising as diverticula of the vasa efferentia and epididymal tubules. In middle age a few pea-sized cysts can usually be felt. Occasionally these cysts become large enough to be a nuisance.

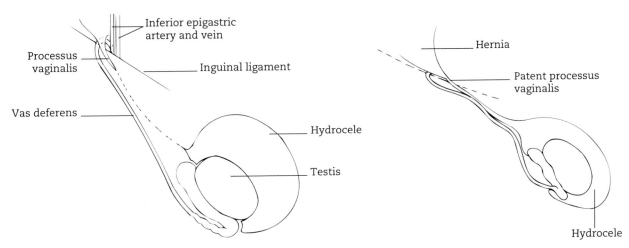

Fig. 22.23 Hydrocele.

Fig. 22.24 Infantile hydrocele.

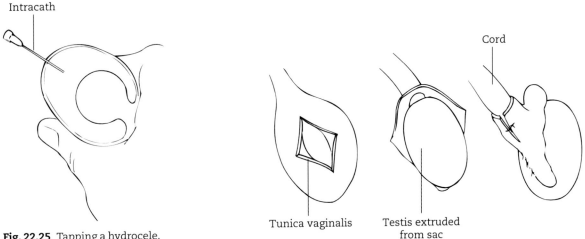

Fig. 22.25 Tapping a hydrocele.

Fig. 22.26 Jaboulay operation for hydrocele.

The swellings are always fluctuant and usually transmit light easily. If aspirated, the fluid often looks opalescent, like lime-water, because a few sperms are present. Occasionally there are so many to make the fluid look like cream. Pregnancy has been reported by injecting these sperms.

The diagnosis is easily confirmed by ultrasound. Treatment is usually unnecessary. Aspiration is usually futile because the cysts fill up again and are always multilocular. Excision of the cysts will often result in a blockage of the vasa efferentia, and should be postponed until the patient has completed his family (Fig. 22.27).

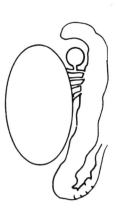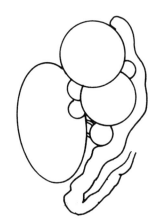

Fig. 22.27 Cysts of the epididymis.

TRAUMA TO THE TESTICLE

The testis is easily injured in sport or at work. Blood collects in the cavity of the tunica vaginalis. The danger is that expansion of the clot may produce pressure-atrophy of the rest of the testis, and for this reason injured testes should all be explored, the clot evacuated, and the rent in the tunica albuginea sewn up (Fig. 22.28).

Testicular tumours are notoriously apt to present after trauma and surgeons must always keep this possibility in mind because an orchiectomy may be needed.

INFLAMMATION OF THE TESTICLE

ACUTE ORCHITIS

Most infections in the testis are caused by viruses, e.g. Coxsackie or mumps. Mumps orchitis only occurs after puberty, when it may be bilateral and the oedema may lead to pressure necrosis and atrophy of the testis. When unilateral it is impossible to distinguish from torsion and therefore demands to be explored. There is some evidence that incision of the tunica albuginea will decompress the testis and prevent atrophy.

ACUTE EPIDIDYMITIS

Bacterial infection finds its way down the vas deferens from the urinary tract to cause acute inflammation. This is seen after operations on the urinary tract especially if a catheter has been left in the urethra. The organisms are usually *Escherichia coli*. Acute epididymitis arising out of the blue may be caused by

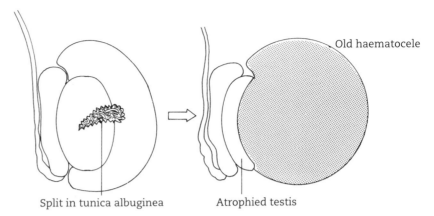

Old haematocele

Split in tunica albuginea   Atrophied testis

Fig. 22.28 Closed injury of the testis: if not evacuated, the clot may cause atrophy of the testis.

Chlamydia trachomatis, which can be identified in fluid aspirated from the epididymis with special culture techniques. Rarely, tuberculosis can cause surprisingly acute symptoms and should be excluded in every acute case where there is no obvious cause for infection such as a recent operation on the urinary tract.

CHRONIC ORCHITIS

Syphilitic gumma of the testis is nowadays a pathological curiosity. Cancer is far more likely and in any event, orchiectomy is probably the right treatment.

Granulomatous orchitis occurs with repeated urinary infections and does not always respond to antibiotics, and usually requires orchiectomy.

CHRONIC EPIDIDYMITIS

Tuberculosis

Blood-borne infection with *Mycobacterium tuberculosis* occurs in the head of the epididymis: urine-borne infection involves the tail along with the vas deferens (Fig. 22.29). The epididymis is knobbly and hard, and there may be nodules along the vas. In late cases a sinus forms to the skin of the scrotum. Rectal ultrasound scannning may show tuberculosis of the prostate and seminal vesicles. The diagnosis and treatment follow the rules for tuberculosis elsewhere (see p. 68). After a full course of treatment a residual mass in the epididymis may have to be removed.

Seminal granuloma

After vasectomy many men have induration in the epididymis caused by an inflammatory response to extravasated sperms. It may respond to prednisolone.

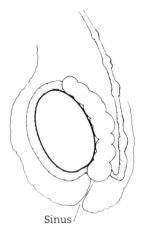

Sinus

Fig. 22.29 Tuberculosis of the epididymis and vas deferens.

ORCHIALGIA

There is a sad group of men who complain of persistent pain in the testicle. Often there has been some previous minor surgical operation, e.g. vasectomy or hydrocelectomy, and pain persists. Careful clinical examination can find nothing wrong. An ultrasound scan is normal. Frequently the testicle is explored and nothing abnormal can be found. Before long the patient seeks a second opinion, and almost inevitably another surgeon will attempt to denervate the testicle. The result is instant relief of pain, for a while, but then it comes back.

Before long the patient has persuaded yet another surgeon to remove the testicle. This is done: the relief of pain is dramatic, for a while, and then it comes back on the other side. It is most important to recognize these unfortunate men because they need help, but from the psychiatrist not the surgeon.

CANCER OF THE TESTIS

AETIOLOGY

Although there are only about 500 new cases in the UK per annum (about 4.5 per 100 000 males), it is the most common cancer in men under the age of 35. It is rare in men of African ancestry both in Africa and elsewhere. It is rare before puberty, and peaks in the early twenties.

One in 10 tumours occurs in association with maldescent of the testis.

PATHOLOGY

Cancer may arise from any of the cell types present in the testis; over 90% arise from germ cells (Fig. 22.30).

Germ cell tumours

Gonadocytes and spermatocytes
These give rise to a spectrum of tumours, from highly anaplastic seminoma which shows nuclear polymorphism and may even stain for human chorionic gonadotrophin, through intermediate types with sheets of cells filled with glycogen that stain for placental alkaline phosphatase (PLAP), to well-differentiated spermatocytic seminoma which seldom metastasize (Fig. 22.31).

Embryonal carcinoma
Here the tissues attempt to form organs, with papillary and glandular elements. They stain for α-fetoprotein (AFP) which betrays the origin of germ cells from the fetal yolk-sac. Pure yolk-sac tumours are occasionally found in infants (Fig. 22.32).

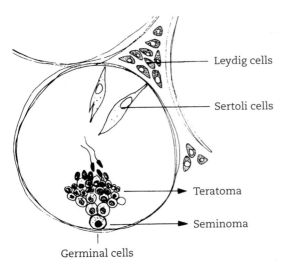

Fig. 22.30 Cellular origin of testicular tumours.

Leydig cells

Sertoli cells

Teratoma

Seminoma

Germinal cells

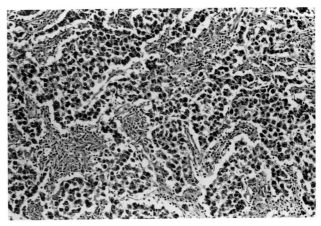

Fig. 22.31 Seminoma.

Epidermoid cyst
A cyst containing mature tissue, mainly skin, is occasionally found. Some of them are possibly benign, but it can take very careful histological examination to distinguish it from teratocarcinoma.

Teratocarcinoma
In this there is a spectrum from the most benign-looking adult tissues, e.g. cartilage and hair, to wildly malignant choriocarcinoma. Of all the possibilities, choriocarcinoma is the worst, spreading rapidly through the bloodstream (Fig. 22.33).

Non-germ cell tumours

Leydig cell tumours
These arise from the Leydig cells that are packed in between the tubules of the testis and normally produce testosterone. They can give rise to precocious puberty.

Sertoli cell tumours
These are very rare, seldom metastasize and cause gynaecomastia.

TNM STAGING OF TESTICULAR TUMOURS

T stage
The T stage is determined only after careful histological examination of the entire testicle (Fig. 22.34).

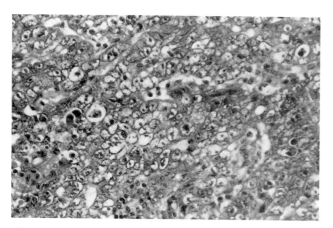

Fig. 22.32 Embryonal carcinoma.

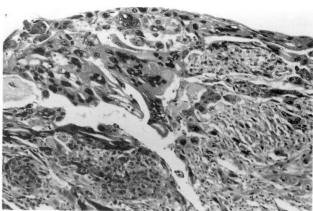

Fig. 22.33 Teratocarcinoma.

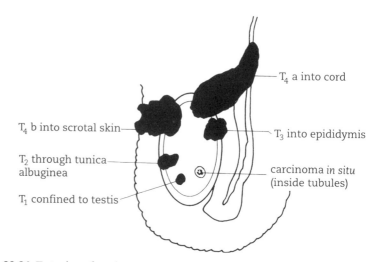

Fig. 22.34 T staging of testis tumours.

N stage

The testis drains to the para-aortic lymph nodes at the level of the origin of the renal arteries, and only later via the cisterna chyli into the thoracic duct and systemic circulation. The nodes are localized by CT scanning (Fig. 22.35).

M stage

Venous spread can occur early if trophoblastic elements are present.

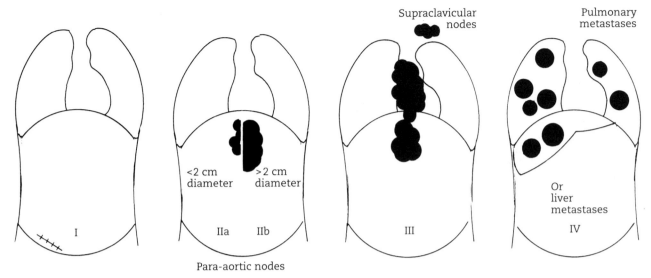

Fig. 22.35 N staging of testis tumours (Royal Marsden Hospital system).

CLINICAL FEATURES

Symptoms

1 *Lump in the testicle*: this can usually be easily felt, is not fluctuant, and is in the body of the testis. The tragedy is that so many young men report this so late (see below).

2 *'Inflammation'*: about 15% have signs of inflammation that are all too often mistaken for epididymitis.

3 *Trauma*: another 15% of men have a history of injury which may lead to loss of valuable time.

4 *Gynaecomastia*: transient swelling of the breasts is common at puberty, but can be due to trophoblastic elements secreting human chorionic gonadotrophin (HCG), which should be measured in every case.

5 *Back pain* in a fit young man should always make you think of metastases from a testicular tumour.

Physical signs

A hard lump is found in the body of the testis. Difficulty arises if the lump is near the epididymis, concealed in the body of the testis, or impossible to feel because of a tense hydrocele (Fig. 22.36). Inflammation can be misleading.

Always examine the breasts for gynaecomastia.

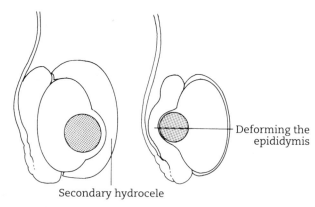

Fig. 22.36 Some testicular tumours are difficult to feel.

INVESTIGATIONS

1 *Ultrasound scan*. This investigation is so quick and painless that it should be performed on every suspicious testicle (Fig. 22.37). Mistakes are rare.

2 *Tumour markers*. Blood is sent for placental alkaline phosphatase (PLAP) which is secreted by gonadocytes, for HCG which is secreted by trophoblastic cells, and AFP secreted by yolk-sac cells. An ordinary 'pregnancy test' is a quick and cheap way of detecting abnormal amounts of HCG.

3 *Exploration of the testicle*. The spermatic cord is clamped at the internal ring before the testicle is delivered: the diagnosis of cancer is usually obvious to the naked eye, but can be verified by frozen section if in doubt. The cord is transected above the clamp (Fig. 22.38).

4 *CT scan*. A CT scan is performed of the chest and abdomen to identify lymph node and pulmonary metastases (Fig. 22.39).

TREATMENT

The treatment of testicular tumours has been revolutionized by platinum-based chemotherapy. Chemotherapy is so unpleasant for the patient that attempts have been made to select out those patients who do not need it, and follow them by surveillance. After many trials this comes down to a small group, excluding all seminomas, any germ cell tumours which have invaded the tissues around the testis, and any that secrete AFP or HCG.

Stage I

Staging retroperitoneal lymph node dissection

This is performed in many centres to identify microscopic metastases with the advantage that removing the lymph nodes may cure those with small volume disease. Where there are larger amounts of tumour present in the lymph nodes,

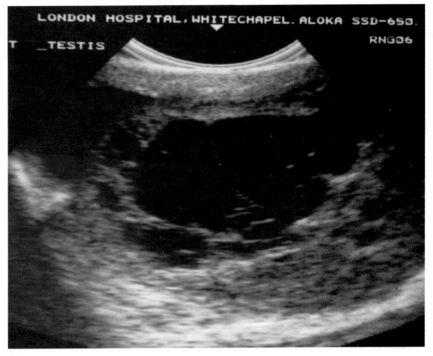

Fig. 22.37 Ultrasound scan of a testicular teratoma. Courtesy of Dr W. Hately.

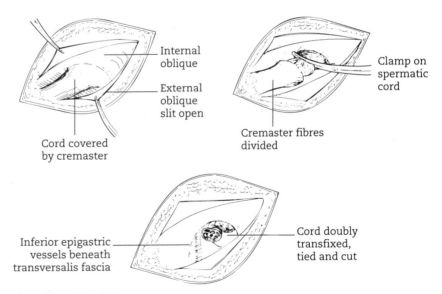

Fig. 22.38 Left orchiectomy.

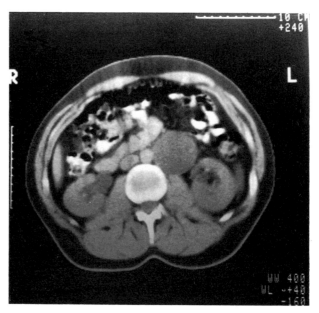

Fig. 22.39 CT scan showing para-aortic mass on the left side of the aorta.

chemotherapy is given afterwards. In most UK centres reliance is placed for staging on CT scanning.

Seminoma
Prophylactic radiation to the retroperitoneal lymph nodes can given 100% cure with stage I seminoma. An identical rate of cure is obtained with a single course of single-agent carboplatin. Surveillance is ruled out by the high rate of relapse.

Other germ cell tumours
Surveillance is reasonable for tumours without invasion of the veins or lymphatics of the testis, without yolk-sac elements, and without undifferentiated elements, but the rate of relapse has made many centres revert to a policy of giving all these men prophylactic platinum-based combination chemotherapy.

Stage II
All patients are given chemotherapy to start with and are then followed carefully.

Stage III
All patients are given as much chemotherapy as they can tolerate: and if a mass remains after two or sometimes three cycles of treatment, it is removed surgically. If the mass of lymph nodes is in the retroperitoneal tissue, this requires careful

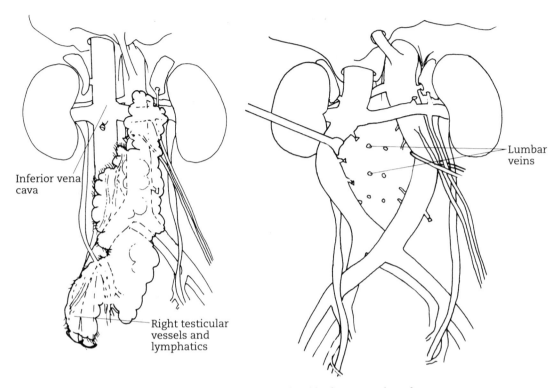

Fig. 22.40 Removal of residual para-aortic nodes.

dissecting of all the tumour off the aorta and inferior vena cava (Fig. 22.40). If the mass is in the mediastinum, the approach is through the chest.

FURTHER READING

Cendron M, Huff DS, Keating MA, Snyder HM, Duckett JW (1993) Anatomical, morphological and volumetric analysis: a review of 759 cases of testicular maldescent. *J Urol* **149**: 570.

Choi SK, Han SW, Lee T (1996) Adolescent varicocele. *Curr Op Urol* **6**: 305.

Cortes D, Thorup JM, Lenz K, Beck BL, Nielsen OH (1995) Laparoscopy in 100 consecutive patients with 128 impalpable testes. *Br J Urol* **75**: 281.

Del Villar RG, Ireland GW, Cass AS (1972) Early exploration in acute testicular conditions. *J Urol* **108**: 887.

Donohue JP, Thornhill JA, Foster RS, Rowland RG, Bihrle R (1993) Retroperitoneal lymphadenectomy for clinical stage A testis cancer (1965–1989): modifications of technique and impact on ejaculation. *J Urol* **149**: 237.

Fenner MN, Roszhart DA, Texter JH (1991) Testicular scanning: evaluating the acute scrotum in the clinical setting. *Urology* **38**: 237.

Friedman NB (1988) Pathology of testicular tumors. In: Skinner DG, Lieskovsky G (eds) *Diagnosis and Management of Genitourinary Cancer*. Philadelphia, WB Saunders, pp. 215–34.

Goldstein M (1992) Methods of vasal occlusion and vasectomy failure. In: Walsh PC (ed.) *Campbell's Urology*, 6th edn. Philadelphia, W.B. Saunders Co. pp. 3123–4.

Hendry WF, A'Hern RP, Hetherington JW, Peckham MJ, Dearnley DP, Horwich A (1993) Para-aortic lymphadenectomy for metastatic non-seminomatous germ cell tumours: prognostic value and therapeutic benefit. *Br J Urol* **71**: 208.

Heyns CF, Hutson JM (1995) Historical review of theories on testicular descent. *J Urol* **153**: 754.

Johnsen SG (1970) Testicular biopsy score count — a method for registration of spermatogenesis in human testis: normal values and results in 335 hypogonadal males. *Hormones* **1**: 1.

Mulhall JP, Albertsen PC (1995) Hemospermia: diagnosis and management. *Urology* **46**: 463.

Philp T, Guillebaud J, Budd D (1984) Complications of vasectomy: review of 16000 patients. *Br J Urol* **56**: 745.

Setchell BP (1978) *The Mammalian Testis*. London, Elek.

Wallace AF (1960) Aetiology of the idiopathic hydrocele. *Br J Urol* **32**: 79.

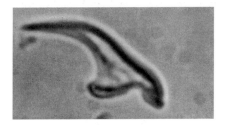

Male Fertility

INVESTIGATION

History and general examination

Gross endocrine deficiencies are usually obvious: the young man who shaves daily and has a normal physique is unlikely to have a deficiency of androgens. Even more rare is it to detect a pituitary tumour that is secreting an excess of prolactin. Corticosteroids taken by athletes may suppress pituitary gonadotrophins. Note any history of previous surgery to the bladder neck or pelvis that may have injured the autonomic nervous system.

Testicles

Very small testes should raise the suspicion of Klinefelter's syndrome (XXY) (Fig. 23.1). Note the presence of a varicocele (see below). Previous surgery for repair of a hernia, or orchiopexy, may suggest damage to the vas deferens. Previous bilateral orchiopexy often, but not always, means that both testicles are not producing sperm.

Semen analysis

Semen is collected by masturbation after 72h abstinence into a clean plastic container.

1 *Volume.* The normal range is from 1 to 8 ml. The most usual cause for a low semen volume is clumsy collection of the specimen.

2 *Sperm density and motility.* Most of the standard methods for measuring sperm density and motility are so inaccurate as to be useless. When the computerized Hamilton–Thorn system is used normal fertility is found with a sperm density as low as 1×10^6/ml provided motility is adequate.

3 *Morphology.* There is very little correlation betwen morphological abnormalities and infertility. Many more are picked up by electron microscopy (Fig. 23.2), but are of doubtful relevance.

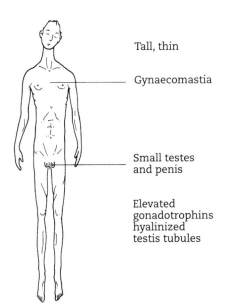

Tall, thin

Gynaecomastia

Small testes
and penis

Elevated
gonadotrophins
hyalinized
testis tubules

Fig. 23.1 Klinefelter's syndrome.

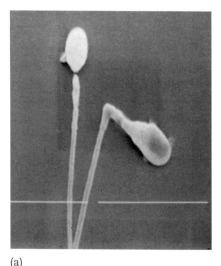 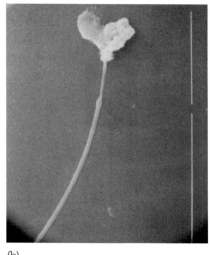

(a)   (b)

Fig. 23.2 Scanning electron microscopy of 'abnormal' morphology of sperms. Courtesy of Mr D.F. Badenoch.

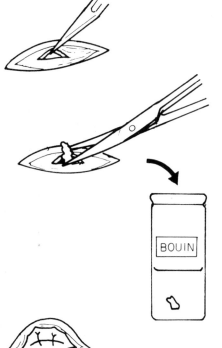

Fig. 23.3 Biopsy of testis.

4 *Antibodies.* Antibodies to the head and tail of the sperm may be found in blood and seminal plasma, and in cervical mucus. These may account for some of the immotile sperms which are sometimes found in a postcoital test.

Luteinizing hormone and follicle-stimulating hormone measurements

A follicle-stimulating hormone (FSH) level greater than 15 mIU/ml means that the tubules are not producing sperms, and for all practical purposes, there is no point in doing a testicular biopsy. If normal it suggests that there may be a blockage somewhere between the testis and the ejaculatory duct.

Testis biopsy

A needle sample is taken from the testis, or a tiny snippet of tubules is taken at open operation (Fig. 23.3). The tissue is put immediately into Bouin's preservative fluid, not ordinary formalin, to avoid distortion of the histology. It is rare for a testis biopsy to show any condition that can be put right by treatment.

TREATMENT

Azoospermia

If the FSH and luteinizing hormone (LH) are elevated, testicular biopsy will add nothing to the diagnosis. If there is any suspicion of Klinefelter's syndrome, a scraping from the mucosa of the cheek is examined cytologically for the Barr body —the index of the extra X chromosome. If a testis biopsy is done and shows maturation arrest (Fig. 23.4), medication with Pergonal may enable completion of the cycle of spermatogenesis. The presence of lymphocytes in the biopsies suggests an immunological problem.

Blockage to the seminal tract may occur from a number of causes. There may have been exposure to mercury in childhood, once a common component of 'teething powders' which paralysed the microcilia in the bronchioles as well as the epididymis.

A blockage in the vas deferens can be demonstrated with a vasogram (Fig. 23.5). The ejaculatory ducts may be obstructed, causing a dilatation of the seminal vesicles which is seen in a transrectal ultrasound scan. Each of these conditions can sometimes be relieved by epididymovasostomy (Fig. 23.6).

Oligozoospermia

When a 'low sperm count' has been reported, the first step must be to check it with a properly validated computerized technique. Because of the errors in the usual methods, claims that any form of treatment has done good must be treated with considerable scepticism. Loose pants and ice packs have had their vogue. Operations on varicoceles, whether they can be seen, or have to be detected by Doppler studies in symptomless men, should be regarded with even more

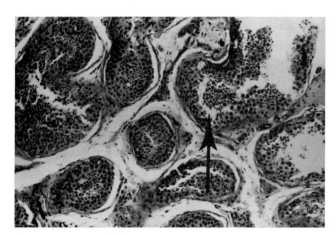

Fig. 23.4 Maturation arrest: the arrow shows immature cells shed into the lumen of the tubule.

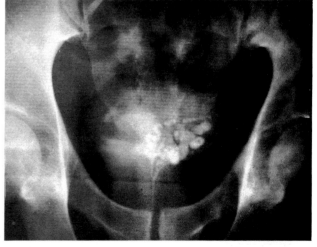

Fig. 23.5 Vasogram showing filling of the vas deferens and seminal vesicle on the left side.

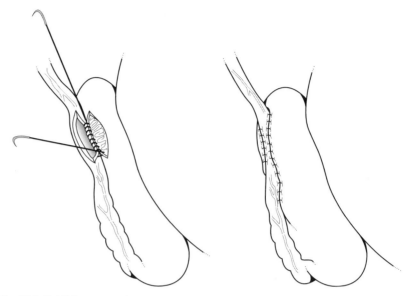

Fig. 23.6 Epididymovasostomy.

scepticism. This is an area which cries out for study of 'evidence-based' surgery (see p. 261).

VASECTOMY

Consent

Both partners must understand that vasectomy is likely to be irreversible. It must also be explained that however carefully the vasa are divided, the ends may grow together. Usually this is detected within the first few months after the vasectomy (early failure) but in something like 1 : 2000 cases it occurs some years later (late failure) and takes place irrespective of what type of operation has been done.

Until all the sperms have disappeared from the ejaculate the couple must continue to use contraceptive precautions.

Because of the risk of medicolegal consequences all these points should be fully discussed, and spelled out on the consent form.

ANAESTHESIA

Vasectomy can be performed under local or general anaesthesia. When there has been previous surgery in the inguinal region or scrotum general anaesthesia may be preferable.

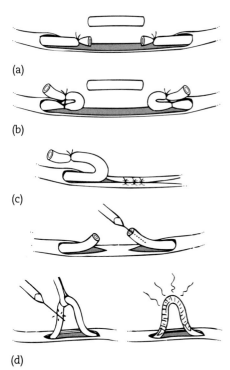

(a)

(b)

(c)

(d)

Fig. 23.7 Variety of methods used in vasectomy in the hope of preventing early or late recanalization.

VASECTOMY

The large number of different techniques in use today shows that none of them is perfect. There is no objective evidence that any one method is superior to another in terms of preventing either early or late reunion.

Usually a small length of vas is removed, and the ends are treated to seal them off in the hope of preventing spontaneous reunion (Fig. 23.7). The ends may be ligated with absorbable or non-absorbable material, metal clips or diathermized. Some surgeons seal one vas, others both. Some surgeons double one, some both ends back. Some stitch the sheath of the vas to interpose a layer of 'fascia' between the two ends. Many do not. Both early and late recurrence has been reported after all of these methods, and it almost certainly takes place more frequently than is generally appreciated: in 10% of one series of men who came up to have their vasectomy reversed it was found that spermatozoa were present in their pre-reversal specimens.

Complications

1 Haematoma is common, from reactionary bleeding from small scrotal veins that go into spasm during the operation and escape notice. A large haematoma is dealt with by early evacuation of the clot and haemostasis. Small collections usually resolve spontaneously.

2 Infection may take place, usually at the site of a skin suture, sometimes in a haematoma.

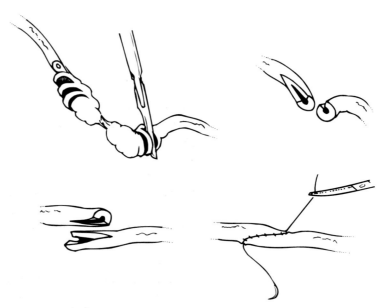

Fig. 23.8 Reversal of vasectomy.

3   Pain in the scrotum. A small number of patients continue to complain of pain in the scrotum for which no cause can be found (see p. 267).

4   Sperm granuloma. Sometimes a sperm granuloma is found at the site of the division of the vas or epididymis to give a typical tender nodular swelling (see p. 267).

REANASTOMOSIS OF THE VAS: 'REVERSAL' OF VASECTOMY

The ends of the vas are found, trimmed back to the lumen, and sewn together (Fig. 23.8). Most surgeons use magnification when performing this operation. Success in terms of sperms finding their way through the anastomosis can be expected in over 80%, but only about 50% will father children. There are many possible reasons for this, including the possible development of autoantibodies during the time that sperms have been obstructed in the epididymis.

FURTHER READING

Ahmed I, Rasheed S, White C, Shaikh NA (1997) The incidence of post-vasectomy chronic testicular pain and the role of nerve stripping (denervation) of the spermatic cord in its management. *Br J Urol* **79**: 269.

Badenoch DF, Moore HDM, Holt WV, Evans PR, Sidhu BS, Evans SJW (1990) Sperm motility, velocity and migration. *Br J Urol* **65**: 204.

Goluboff ET, Stifelman MD, Fisch H (1995) Ejaculatory duct obstruction in the infertile male. *Urology* **45**: 925–31.

Hendry WF, Levison DA, Parkinson MC, Parslow JM, Royle MG (1990) Testicular obstruction: clinico-pathological studies. *Ann Roy Coll Surg Engl* **72**: 396.

Jecquier AM, Ukombe EB (1983) Errors inherent in the performance of a routine semen analysis. *Br J Urol* **55**: 434.

Holt W, Watson P, Curry M, Holt C (1994) Reproducibility of computer-aided semen analysis: comparison of five different systems used in a practical workshop. *Fertil Steril* **62**: 1277.

Ohl DA, Naz RK (1995) Infertility due to antisperm antibodies. *Urology* **46**: 591–602.

Smith JC (1996) Long-term complications of vasectomy. *Curr Op Urol* **6**: 344.

van Steirtegham A, Verheyen G, Tournaye H, Devroey P (1996) Assisted reproductive technology by intracytoplasmic sperm injection in male-factor infertility. *Curr Op Urol* **6**: 333.

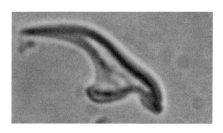

Glossary of Urological Eponyms and Jargon

agenesis. Greek α plus γένεσις (creation)

albumen. Latin, egg-white

allantois. Greek αλλας (sausage)

Alport, Cecil (1880–1959) South African physician

ampulla. Latin, a flask

aplasia. Greek α plus πλασσειν (to form)

balanitis. Greek βαλανος (the glans penis)

Barr, Murray (1908) Contemporary Canadian anatomist

Behçet, Hulúsi (1889–1948) Turkish dermatologist

Bellini, Lorenzo (1643–1704) Anatomist of Pisa

Bence-Jones, Henry (1814–73) Physician, London

Benedict, Stanley Rossiter (1884–1936) Biochemist, New York

Bertin, Exupère Joseph (1712–81) Associate anatomist, Academy of Sciences, Paris

Bilharz, Theodor Maximilian (1825–62) German physician working in Cairo who discovered *Schistosoma haematobium*

Boari, Achille (b. 1894) Italian urologist

Bonney, W.F. Victor (1872–1953) Gynaecologist, Middlesex Hospital, London

bougie. French, candle (the best wax came from Bujiyah in Algeria)

Bouin, Paul (1870–1962) Histologist of Strasbourg: devised fixative containing picric and acetic acids as well as formalin

Bowman, Sir William (1816–92) Ophthalmic surgeon, London

Brucella. Microorganisms discovered by Sir William Bruce (1855–1931), British surgeon

Buck, Gordon (1807–77) Surgeon, New York

Burch, J.C. American gynaecologist

Buschke, Abraham (1868–1943) German pathologist

calix. Greek κάλιξ (cup). Often confused with Graeco-Latin κάλυξ (the leaves covering the bud of a flower), and incorrectly written as calyx

Camper, Peter (1772–89) Physician of Amsterdam

cannula. Latin (canna, a reed)

catheter. Greek καθετηρ, καθεμη (to send down)

Chlamydia. Greek χλάμυς (cloak)

chordée. Painful curvature of the penis: French *cordée*

clitoris. Greek (κλειτορίς)

Colles, Abraham (1773–1843) Professor of Surgery in Dublin

Conn, Jerome W. (1907) American physician

Cowper, William (1666–1709) Surgeon of London

creatinine. Greek κρέας (flesh: product of catabolism of protein)

Crohn, Burrill B. (1884–1983) Gastroenterologist, New York

Cushing, Harvey (1869–1939) Neurosurgeon of Boston

de la Peyronie, François (1678–1747) Surgeon of Paris

Denonvilliers, Charles Pierre (1802–72) Surgeon of Paris

detrusor. Latin (detrudere, to push down)

diabetes. Latin (syphon)

dilate. Latin, dilatare: *di-* plus *latus* (wide) hence dilatation (dilation is incorrect)

Doppler, Christian Johann (1803–53) Austrian physicist

Ducrey, Augusto (1860–1940) Dermatologist of Rome

Dupuytren, Baron Guillaume (1777–1835) French surgeon and pathologist

dysplasia. Greek δύς (difficult, bad, etc.) plus πλασσειν (formation)

Echinococcus. Greek ἐχῖνος (hedgehog), κόκκος (grain, seed)

ectopic. Greek εκτώπος (displaced)

enuresis. Greek ἐνουρειν (incontinence): usually applied today to bed-wetting

epididymis. Greek ἐπι plus διδυμοι (twins—testes)

epispadias. Greek ἐπι plus σπάδον (a rent or tear)

Escherich, Theodor (1857–1911) Paediatrician of Munich

exstrophy. Greek ἐξστρεφειν (to turn inside out)

Falloppius, Gabriel (1523–62) Anatomist of Padua: favourite pupil of Vesalius

fasciculata. Latin *fasciculus* (packet, bundle)

Foley, Frederic Eugene Basil (1891–1966) Urologist of Minneapolis-St Paul

fossa. Latin (ditch)

fraenum, fraenulum. Latin (bridle)

fundus. Bottom

Gimbernat, Don Manuel Louis (1734–1816) Anatomist, Barcelona

Giraldes, Joachim (1808–75) Professor of Surgery, Paris

glomerulus. Latin (little ball)

Goodpasture, Ernest William (1886–1960) American pathologist

Grawitz, Paul Albert (1850–1932) Pathologist of Greifswald

gubernaculum. Latin (rudder; described by John Hunter, sometimes called Hunter's gubernaculum)

Hartnup. Surname of English family in whom the disease was first described

Henle, Freidrich (1809–85) Anatomist of Berlin

Henoch, E. (1820–1910) Paediatrician, Berlin

hilum. Latin (eye of seed or bean, hence applied to kidney)

Hounsfield, Sir Godfrey Newbold (b. 1919) Nobel laureate, inventor of CT and MRI scanners

Hunner, Guy Leroy (1868–1951) Gynaecologist, Johns Hopkins, Baltimore

hyaline. Greek ὑαλου (glass)

hydatid. Greek ὑδῶρ (drop of water)

hydrocele. Greek υδῶρ (water) plus κήλη (swelling; often misspelt hydrocoele from confusion with κόιλιακος meaning belly)

insipidus. Latin (tasteless; diabetes insipidus, the urine does not taste sweet)

Jaboulay, Mathieu (1860–1913) Surgeon of Lyons

Jensen, Carl Oluf (1864–1934) Pathologist of Copenhagen

Katayama, Kunika (1886–1931) Japanese Physician

Klinefelter, Harry Fitch (b. 1912) Contemporary radiologist, Massachusetts General Hospital

Leydig, Franz von (1821–1908) Anatomist of Bonn

litho-. Greek λιθος (stone), hence tripsy, from τριβειν (to crush), τομή (cut), λάπαξειν (to evacuate)

Littré, Alexis (1658–1726) Anatomist of Paris

Löwenstein, Ernst pathologist of Vienna

malacoplakia. Greek μαλακός and πλακος (plaque)

Marshall, Victor F. (1913–1996) Urologist, New York Memorial Hospital

meatus. Latin (passage or channel)

mellitus. Latin *mel* (honey, honey-sweet; diabetes mellitus, urine tastes sweet)

micturition. Latin (urinate), derived from *mingere* (to mix). Originally meant frequency

Millin, Terence (1903–1980) Irish urologist working in London

Morgagni, Giovanni Battista (1682–1771) Anatomist of Padua

Müller, Johannes (1801–58) Physiologist of Berlin

navicularis. Latin (shaped like a boat)

Neisser, Albert Ludwig Siegmund (1855–1916) Dermatologist, Breslau

nephro-. Greek νέφρον. Nephrosis, -οσις (condition), nephritis, -ητις (inflammation)

nexus. Latin (tying together, as in connect, etc.)

nocturia. Latin *nocte* (night: passing abnormal amounts of urine in the night)

Page, I. Harriet Contemporary American physician, Cleveland clinic

pampiniform. Latin *pampinus* (tendril)

Papanicolaou, George N. (1883–1962) Greek pathologist working in New York

papilla. Latin (nipple)

papilloma. Latin (nipple) plus Greek ωμα (tumour)

Petit, Jean Louis (1674–1760) Parisian surgeon, elected to the Royal Society of London

Pfannenstiel, Hermann Johann (1862–1909) Gynaecologist, Breslau

polyuria. Greek πόλυ (much) plus ὀυρια (passing much urine)

posthitis. Greek πόσθε (foreskin)

Potter, Edith Louise (b. 1901) American perinatal pathologist

Queyrat, L. (b. 1911) Dermatologist, Paris

Randall, Alexander (1883–1930) Urologist, Philadelphia

Raz, Shlomo Contemporary American urologist, UCLA

Rehn, Ludwig (1849–1930) Surgeon, Frankfurt

reticularis. Latin (net-like)

Rovsing, N.T. (1862–1927) Professor of Surgery, Copenhagen

Sachse, Hans Contemporary German urologist

Scarpa, Antonio (1747–1832) Anatomist, Pavia

Schistosoma. Greek σχιστω (split) plus σωμα (body)

Schönlein, Johann L. (1793–1864) German physician

Scott, F. Brantley Contemporary American urologist

Scribner, Belding H. (b. 1921) Contemporary American nephrologist

Sertoli, Enrico (1842–1910) Anatomist, Pavia

Shy–Drager, Milton G. Shy (1919–1967), Glen A. Drager (b. 1917) American neurologists

spermatozoa. Greek σπερμα (seed) plus σωμα (body)

Stamey, Thomas A. Contemporary American Urologist, Stanford, California

strangury. Greek στράγξ (drop squeezed out) plus ουπον (slow and painful urination)

teratoma. Greek τέρας (monster) plus ομα (swelling)

testis. Latin (witness)

Treponema. Greek τρεπειν (turn), νεμα (thread)

Trichomonas. Greek θριξ (hair) plus μονος (one; though it has three to five hairs)

trocar. French *trois carrés* (three sharp edges)

urethra. Greek ουρηθρα

utriculus. Latin (small bag)

varicocele. Latin *varus* (bent) plus Greek κήλη (swelling)

vas. Latin (a vessel)

verumontanum. Latin *veru* (a spit) *montanum* (mountainous) *vesicle.* Latin (a little bladder)

von Brunn, A. (1841–95) Professor of Anatomy, Gottingen

von Fehling, Hermann Christian (1812–85) German chemist

vulva. Latin (a wrapper)

Whitaker, Robert H. (b. 1939) Contemporary urologist and anatomist, Cambridge

Wilms, Max (1867–1918) Surgeon, Heidelberg (nephroblastoma had previously been described by Rance in 1814)

Wolff, Kaspar Friedrich (1733–94) German anatomist, working in St Petersburg

xanthogranuloma. Greek ξανθός (yellow)

Index